Listening to Less-Heard Voices:

Developing Counsellors' Awareness

CW01497057

Listening to Less-Heard Voices:

Developing Counsellors' Awareness

Edited by

Peter Madsen Gubi

University of Chester Press

First published 2015
by University of Chester Press
University of Chester
Parkgate Road
Chester CH1 4BJ

Printed and bound in the UK by the
LIS Print Unit
University of Chester
Cover designed by the
LIS Graphics Team
University of Chester

The introduction and editorial material
© University of Chester, 2015
The individual chapters
© the respective authors, 2015

All Rights Reserved
No part of this publication may be reproduced, stored in a
retrieval system or transmitted in any form or by any means
without the prior permission of the copyright owner, other
than as permitted by current UK copyright legislation or
under the terms and conditions of a recognised copyright
licensing scheme

A catalogue record for this book is available from the British
Library

ISBN 978-1-908258-23-6

To Amanda Boxer, Alan West
and Avril Davies

CONTENTS

CONTRIBUTORS

Revd Dr Peter Madsen Gubi, PhD, MTh, MA, MA, MA, BEd, MBACP (Reg Snr Accred), FRSA, FHEA, is Senior Lecturer in Counselling at the University of Chester, and Minister of Dukinfield Moravian Church. He is a Counsellor, Supervisor and Spiritual Director in Private Practice, having worked as a Counsellor Trainer and Principal Lecturer in Counselling and Psychotherapy at the University of Central Lancashire, and as a Counsellor in various Education, Voluntary Sector and Primary Care settings. He has a research interest in Spirituality and Counselling, and has researched and published extensively in this field. His books include *Prayer in Counselling and Psychotherapy: Exploring a hidden meaningful dimension* (2008), and *Spiritual Accompaniment and Counselling: Journeying with psyche and soul* (2015).

Kathryn Hackland, BSc (Hons), MA, MBACP, has a background in genetic counselling and is currently working as a Person-Centred Counsellor in an NHS primary care setting.

Leana Hughes, BA (Hons) Psych, MA, MBACP, is a Counsellor in a GP surgery.

Christine Hurst, BSc (Hons) Psych, MA, MBACP, has a special interest in working with women. She currently offers Person-Centred Counselling at a women's centre in the North West of England.

Jennifer Jane Johnson, BA (Hons), PGCE, MA, MBACP, has thirty years' experience working in education and currently works as a Counsellor in a GP practice, and as a

Volunteer Listener for Samaritans. Particular interests include anxiety, depression, adverse life experiences and resilience.

Dr Vida Kennedy, MA, PhD, MBACP, initially trained as a researcher with particular interest in neurology and palliative care for around fifteen years. She has worked with clients that have experienced sexual abuse and currently works as a School Based Counsellor in the North Wales area.

Ann Todd, BA (Hons), MA, MBACP, works as a Counsellor for a small charitable organization. She has a special interest in psychological trauma.

Eleanor Warman, MA, MBACP, works as a Bereavement Counsellor at The Hospice of the Good Shepherd in Backford, near Chester, offering support to clients pre- and post-bereavement, and also works with Cruse Bereavement Care.

ACKNOWLEDGEMENTS

This book is the result of team work, and so it is right to acknowledge, with gratitude, the supervision input of Dr Rita Mintz, Dr Tony Parnell, Dr Valda Swinton and Dr Paul Wagg, from the Division of Counselling and Psychotherapy, within the Department of Social and Political Sciences, at the University of Chester; to acknowledge the support of the families, friends, and colleagues of the chapter authors, and the valuable contributions of the research participants, without whom none of this could have happened. We are particularly grateful for the intensive work of Dr Sarah Griffiths of the University of Chester Press, in bringing this book to fruition.

INTRODUCTION

Peter Madsen Gubi

Much of the recent research that is published in the academic journals on Counselling and Psychology is increasingly quantitative, and largely centred on establishing efficacy and outcome, rather than reflecting on ways of understanding process, in order to meet the political agenda of funders and commissioners of services. It is, therefore, largely (and perhaps boringly) statistical in nature, and doesn't really reflect much of the therapeutic encounter that is probably of most interest to Counsellors – who, by their nature and motivation, are people-persons who are interested in the rich variety of human experiencing (or lived-experience). Excluded from many of the journals are the minority voices of some individuals who do not 'fit into' the way of the majority (or that which has come to define 'normal experiencing'); because, for funding purposes, services have to be best suited to, and be of best value for, the majority. Yet, the emotional needs of some do not always fit with what is best for the majority, but still their voices are of worth, and to be equally valued, and certainly reflected in the literature; or else our profession, and the services that we offer, become poorer and less well-informed. Whilst research is designed to inform best practice and increase understanding, there is less in-depth research published about human experiencing that relates to issues that are 'on the edge' of the professions of Counselling, Psychotherapy and Psychology, yet which are nevertheless 'central' for those people who experience such issues. Theirs are less-heard voices in the literature. The structure of academic journals does not lend itself to being the best forum for qualitative research which, by its very nature,

1

tends to be wordier as it deals with phenomena, rather than be able to be represented through succinct patterns of numeracy (i.e. statistics). Such research doesn't fit neatly into a 5,000 word article without severely editing much valuable material. Whilst some attempts have been made to engage with new researchers, much of what is still published in the journals is from university-employed 'academics' (like myself), rather than from practitioners at the 'coal-face'. 'Academics' are often the ones with the skills to conduct, and disseminate the results of, such projects, and are those who give the journals (and therefore the research and the profession) political credibility and validity – but this comes with the loss of some valuable, and interesting, research that is conducted at practitioner level. This, arguably, is more important to be aware of, and to be informed by, because they are the people doing the transformative work; and their voices, and those of their clients, need to be heard in the literature.

It is therefore refreshing to host this book which disseminates some interesting research, that comes from a place of passion within the researchers, and which is aimed at informing Counsellors about aspects of human experiencing that are not written about much (if at all) in the Counselling-related literature. The title of this book, *Listening to Less-Heard Voices: Developing counsellors' awareness*, reflects this. Each of the chapters in this book comes from research that has been undertaken for a Master of Arts degree in Clinical Coun-selling at the University of Chester. They are all qualitative pieces of distinction standard. They were undertaken to satisfy the deeply held questions and curiosities that arose from the researchers' experiencing. I believe that it is from this place of questioning and curiosity that the best research is motivated and formulated. Each chapter is written by those that some might consider to be unseasoned researchers, who are first-and-foremost practitioners, and who because of that, bring a fresh perspective to the topic that each has studied. Theirs are not voices that are currently heard much (if at all) in the Counselling literature; yet, they have something very worthwhile to contribute to professional dialogue. The format of this book, rather than that of the academic journals, allows a fuller expression of their voices, and those of their participants (inappropriately called 'the thick data'), to be heard; and it is a privilege to host such a range of voices, and experiences, in this book.

Research choices

Another reason for hosting these pieces of research under one cover, is that they all (coincidentally) use Interpretative Phenomenological Analysis (IPA) as their research methodology for analysing the data. Rather than spend wordage in each chapter explaining the methodology, a brief summary of the main points of IPA is presented here. The aim of IPA is to explore, in detail, participants' views of the topic that is under investigation (Smith et al. 2009). It is a phenomenological approach, in that it is concerned with personal perception rather than with the formation of objective statement. It is a method that seeks an insider's perspective, but which takes account of the fact that the researcher's own perceptions are needed to make sense of the other's world through a process of interpretative activity. Therefore, it is the researcher's role to comment on, and make sense of, the participant's activity and opinion. IPA is a bricolage of established approach and methodology, in that it brings together a phenomenological approach and a symbolic interactionism approach, whilst using research instruments and methods of analysis that are commonly found in discourse analysis and thematic analysis. The philosophical paradigm on which IPA is based, is that it is not necessary to go beyond the verbal statement to understand underlying cognitions or to predict the relational dimension between verbal statement and behaviour. Instead, IPA attempts to value the perception and meaning that is attributed to an object, event, or experience, whilst recognizing that meaning can only be obtained through a process of interpretative activity. It is a dynamic process that is complicated by the researcher's own conceptions. The method of analysis is creative, not prescriptive. It relies on a method of making sense of the data through the coding of themes and sub-themes, and the seeking of connections. It is important that the researcher's bias does not distort the selective process of the categorization of themes. Initial themes can be governed by the prompts that are used at the interviewing stage. However, at the transcribing stage, it is important for the richness of the data to determine the emerging themes and categorization, and for the researcher to be led by that process rather than dictate it. Once a master list of themes has emerged, the researcher is then required to be selective towards the emerging sub-themes, with the selectivity dependent on the parameters of the research and the relevance of emerging sub-themes to the research topic. At the writing-up stage of the research, the shared themes, patterns, connections and tensions are translated and woven into a narrative account that details the interesting and essential things about the participants' responses, and the researcher's interpretative analysis of them. This data can be presented in a variety of ways (e.g. diagrammatically to detail the relationships and/or conflicts between emerging themes; or as a narrative that is comprised of the respondents' comments that are interpretatively analysed). However, at this stage of weaving the tapestry that is the narrative, it is important for the unique nature of each participant's experience to emerge; and throughout, the participants' voices are heard in the rich (or thick) data.

Ethical awareness

As each research project was undertaken within the Division of Counselling and Psychotherapy at the University of Chester, it was subject to the rigorous procedure of ethical approval by the University's Research Ethics Committee. Every effort was made to protect the participants from harm, to seek their consent at various stages of the research, to protect their right to withdraw without prejudice, to support them if anything emotional was stirred up within them because of the research process, to maintain the confidentiality of their identities, and to maintain the security of their data.

The structure of each chapter

Each chapter has been edited, and formatted, in such a way as to offer a cohesive and homogeneous presentation that enables each: to set the scene for the research; to establish the research project in published literature that has been searched for, and accessed, through various academic search-engines; to introduce the participants and the questions asked of them in semi-structured interviews; to present the findings; to enable a reflexive and critical discussion of the findings in the light of the published literature; and finally to conclude.

Introducing each chapter

In Chapter One, Leana Hughes seeks to explore tattoo narratives as an alternative approach to understanding a client's phenomenological sense of self. Her research gives some understanding of why some clients choose to immortalize significant life events with tattoos, and attach personal meaning to them.

In Chapter Two, Kathryn Hackland explores the impact of Person-Centred training on important friendships. Her data shows that friendships are impacted both negatively, but largely positively, by Person-Centred Counsellor training. Emerging themes include notions such as outgrowth, and the collision of worlds, as Counsellors try to integrate changes into their lives. Counsellors become enriched by new ways of relating, and seek this out from their friendships. The friendship landscape necessarily changes as they consciously engage with the core conditions.

In Chapter Three, Jennifer Jane Johnson has explored people's lived-experience of their relationships with companion animals. Of particular interest were the everyday aspects of the relationship. The findings are generally consistent with other research in the area, in that they show the central role that companion animals play in the participants' lives, and the uplifting, life-enhancing qualities that they bestow. Each participant had come through difficult times in their lives, with a sense that their companion animal relationship had been restorative, sustaining and motivating. An additional interest was to discover if people felt inhibited in speaking about the depth of the bond; such a finding could be a useful factor for Counsellors to consider when working with clients. The study confirms that, for Counsellors, an appreciation of the important contribution of pets to happiness and well-being could add a significant dimension to understanding a client's world. It is suggested that the human–animal bond merits attention in Counselling training, research and practice.

Introduction

In Chapter Four, Christine Hurst explores women's lived-experience of non-physical abuse within an intimate heterosexual relationship, when there is no physical abuse. Her research shows that the most salient feature of emotional abuse is its insidious nature, with many types of emotionally abusive behaviour appearing socially acceptable. Women can experience non-physical abuse (NPA) for years without recognizing their partner's behaviour as abusive. When there is no overt abuse, Counsellors may not be aware of the presence of NPA within the relationship. The study found that NPA was unrecognized and unseen. The effects of those who experience NPA included: self-blame, a loss of confidence, and a loss of a sense of self. The findings were largely consistent with other research into NPA.

In Chapter Five, Ann Todd explores mothers' experiences of the impact of traumatic birth. Her research found that mothers experienced feelings of fear, shock and being out of control during the trauma. Coping mechanisms of dissociation and repression were reported. Feelings of failure, anger, inadequacy and depression featured post-partum. The trauma also impacted on marital relationships, mother–baby bonding, attachment behaviour and decisions about future pregnancies. Post-traumatic growth was also a feature of the impact of traumatic birth.

In Chapter Six, Eleanor Warman investigates the experiences of Person-Centred Counsellors who have worked with clients who have presented with Complicated Grief. Her results indicate that working as a Bereavement Counsellor impacts on the self of the Counsellor in positive ways (such as personal satisfaction and intellectual stimulation), and in negative ways (such as feelings of self-doubt about competence, or the emotional risks of working with themes of death and loss). Ongoing self-care (monitoring and attendance) was deemed vital, with team work viewed as a gift, and supervision referenced as critical. The relationship became a tool in the work, and the study found these Person-Centred participants shied away from labelling grief, were not panicked by suicidal inclinations in clients, felt that bereavement is not a linear process, and that sitting with difficult emotions was part of their job.

Finally, in Chapter Seven, Vida Kennedy investigates the role of mother-tongue in counselling Welsh clients, and within the therapeutic relationship. Her study found that all participants described mother-tongue as an important aspect of counselling, and of the counselling relationship. The results demonstrated that the more familiar a language is to the client, the easier it is to talk about personal experiences and emotions. It also highlighted the role that language plays in the client's identity and culture, and that it is important for the therapist to accept, and understand, the client's background, and their struggle to communicate, in order to create a facilitative relationship, and a safe environment for counselling. The study found that aspects, such as searching for the right word, or having meaning get lost in translation, acted as barriers to counselling. Language was used to create closeness, or distance, to an issue, and being bilingual allows for flexibility and choice.

Who this book is for

This book is written to disseminate research to Counsellors and Psychotherapists – those who are qualified and those who are in training – in order to develop their awareness of the issues that are covered in each chapter. However, the insights that the researches provide are applicable, and will be of interest, to anyone who is interested in understanding people better, and those who are involved in people-work –

where the accompaniment of those in emotional difficulty is paramount (e.g. Social Workers, Pastoral Care workers, Chaplains, Clergy, Clinical and Counselling Psychologists, Nurses, Prison Wardens, etc.).

CHAPTER ONE
THE TATTOOED CLIENT:
SYMBOLIC REPRESENTATIONS OF SELF

Leana Hughes

Introduction

Rogers (1961) reminds us of the unique opportunity we have, as Counsellors, to form intimate therapeutic relationships with clients from all walks of life. We encounter individuals that differ from us in age, race, gender, faith, values, social backgrounds and life experiences. Clients employ a variety of narratives to share who they are in life and in the counselling room. Giddens (1991) contends that the 'identity' of the self is not a stagnant generic phenomenon, but something that has to be routinely created and sustained in the reflexive activities of the individual' (Giddens 1991, p. 52). The paramount part of our training and personal development as Counsellors is to explore our own attitudinal perceptions, preconceived ideas and limitations to working with individuals that identify themselves differently to ourselves. I might not understand why anyone would want to have their tongue surgically split to give the appearance of a snake tongue, whereas I will adorn my own body with tattoos. Paradoxically, my mother cannot see why on earth I would want to mutilate my body with permanent ink, but she wears earrings in pierced ears. As Counsellors we need to have unconditional positive regard and a non-judgemental attitude to all facets of our client (Merry 2002).

The purpose of this chapter, therefore, is to bring an explicit and new conversation to counselling research. Body modification is an ever-expanding form of expression. My focus fell on the use of tattoos as an extension of a reflexive self-concept. This chapter is written to inform Counsellors on how body art or body modification creates dialogue that is capable of producing the richest discourse and phenomenological exploration of a person's idea of identity, socio-culture and self-expression. It illuminates the potential for a missed opportunity that talking about a client's tattoo can offer. The understanding of semiotics in tattoo design might not be new to the tattooed client, but it can be a fascinating and alternative dimension for a Counsellor to work with.

I have a great personal interest in tattoos. I carry a back piece that reflects transitions in my own life. This study developed from my own reflexivity on the meaning that I attach to my growing tattoo. From speaking about my tattoo to others, I came to understand that many tattooed people see their tattoos as part of their identity narrative. My rationale for examining 'tattoo narratives' (DeMello 2000; Kosut 2000) was to connect the tattoo community with the Counsellor that might not have contact with many tattooed people – who might not understand why a person would have a tattoo, or who have never considered using a client's tattoo as a way of making psychological contact. Clients in everyday life explore a variety of topics in the counselling room – grief and mourning; transition; examining self and identity. Tattooed people in everyday life talk about similar topics, but through non-verbal embodied semiotics. This study sheds light on why a person would choose to carry a permanent reminder of life events or losses. If our identity narrative is informed by our sense of self, a tattoo could be explained as a visual presentation of that self-identity.

It is evident that there is a lack of UK-based literature on the contemporary subject matter of linking tattoo narratives with the understanding of personal meaning-making and phenomenology. Counselling literature does not cover the topic of body modification as a form of self-concept exploration. Available UK-based qualitative research on tattoos place focus on a host of different avenues of identity theory. Patterson and Schroeder's (2010) focus of inquiry related tattoos to the understanding of embodied identity within Consumer Culture Theory (CCT). Interestingly, my research does highlight similar findings to the work of John Follett's (2009) investigation of permanence in terms of tattoo consumption and identity creation, although Follett's work also relates his findings in terms of CCT. My interest lay with the lived-experience of the participant's sense of self and the utility a tattoo plays in that identity construction.

Conducting this research reminded me of our ability as humans to change and construct our self-concept as we grow and develop. Identity narratives flow out of our sense of who we are and how we experience ourselves in everyday life. Heidegger viewed the self as a human construction – a way of being in the world. Without an interpretive stance, or a context in which we exist, there is no consciousness (Smith et al. 2009) to our experience of who we are, and in turn cuts off our identity narrative, sense of self and (for some) tattoo narrative. And as we are in constant flow, we have the opportunity to rewrite our identity narrative all the time (Rogers 1961). It was a privilege to immerse myself into four individuals' tattoo narrative.

This research is about creating the potential of expanding identity narrative, by exploring phenomenological tattoo narratives (DeMello 2000). The purpose of this study was to create a new or alternative window of opportunity in making psychological contact with a tattooed client (Merry 2002). The understanding of semiotics in tattoo design might not be new to the tattooed client, but it can be a fascinating and alternative dimension for a Counsellor to work with if they choose to. This study is relevant as it can inform Counsellors on how body art or body modification creates dialogue, capable of producing the richest discourse and phenomenological exploration of a person's idea of identity, socio-culture and self-expression.

What the literature says

As there is already a vast amount of research and reading material on the history of tattoos, and as my interest focuses on modern day tattoo wearers, I will only give a brief historical overview post 1980. DeMello (2000) accurately summed up the shift that happened post 1980 in North America as the *Tattoo Renaissance*. Tattoos were mostly worn by the lower-class, deviant, sailors or tribes (Pitts 2003; Klesse 2000). The nineties saw a cultural shift to mainstream middle-class America. Tattoos became a symbol for counter-culture or resistance to middle-class values (DeMello 2000). The skin became a canvas for a more artistic form of personal expression and revolution. Removed from the traditional 'old school' tattoo community, this new wave of middle-class tattoo wearers created a discourse among themselves, communicating the motivations behind their designs and what these tattoos meant to them. DeMello contends that new meaning is created through the sharing of tattoo narratives. It creates an opportunity to share and provide a framework for understanding their tattoos, their community and themselves, producing the contemporary tattoo community of today (DeMello 2000).

Evidence seems to suggest that most participants would bring identity narratives of individualism, especially for people wearing custom tattoos (e.g. DeMello 2000; Turner 2000). The wearer might feel separate from their immediate 'neighbour', especially if their tattoo is a unique piece of art and their 'neighbour' carries no tattoos themself, but complete individualism is questioned due to the wearer's affiliation to the wider tattoo community. Moerier et al. (2011) would argue that this affiliation to a group serves as a source of identification for the individual. Muggleton (1995) found that few contemporary tattoo wearers linked their tattoos to membership of a specific subculture, even suggesting 'label rejection' as a way to sidestep being perceived as part of a group (p. 4). Individuality also comes into question for wearers of traditional tattoos like swallows, anchors or pin-up girls – a style that has seen a surge in popularity in recent years, creating a subgenre to traditional tattoos termed 'Neo-traditional'. As my study is idiographic in nature, my intention is not to make any claims or take any stances between traditional versus new style of tattooing, but instead to highlight areas of previous research in addressing tattoos as pieces of individualism or collectivism. DeMello takes tattoo community studies a step further by reporting on the role of the tattoo artist and tattoo magazines in 'controlling the borders of community' and therefore elevating their own reputations as artists (DeMello 2000, p. 124), clearly separating members into higher- or lower-status groups.

Tattoo narratives can also connect with the discourse of spirituality, some describing the experience of being tattooed as spiritualistic or ritualistic (Goode and Vail 2008), especially among the modern primitive community. Originating in the 1970s in California, Modern Primitives is a subculture community that celebrates their sense of freedom to choose their identities, bodies and cultural affiliations (Pitts 2003; Klesse 2000). This group largely consists of the body modification community who 'responds to primal urges to *do something* with their bodies' (Fakir Musafar, cited in Klesse 2000, p. 15). This could be any form of *Body Play* (e.g. by fire, by suspension or penetration) that creates a ritualistic, spiritual experience, or in some cases, erotic experience offered by penetration. In the context of my study, I am discussing the spiritual connection offered by penetration through tattooing. Evidence seems to suggest a counter argument to the idea of spiritual connection and reasoning behind *Body Play* (Eubanks 1996; DeMello 2000). Eubanks contested Modern Primitives' adoption of ritual form of body modification as a 'blatant disregard for the history and the context of the symbols and practices involved' (Eubanks 1996, p. 74). DeMello described it as a form of elitism in contemporary tattoo culture – a way to distance the wearer from working-class associations (Pitts 2003).

The second point of argument is the Modern Primitives' view of changeable identity. According to Pitts, this is questionable because of our deep entrenchment in categories of gender, race, citizenship and sexuality (Pitts 2003; Klesse 2000). Friedman (1994) and Giddens (1991) contend this modernist viewpoint of choosing and changing identity by stating that it has done nothing more than create a 'widespread subjective feeling of alienation', describing individuals as being separated from their embeddedness of anything cohesive and meaningful (Friedman, cited in Klesse 2000, p. 23). Patterson and Schroeder's work on tattoos and consumer culture theory considers the tension between considerations of 'consumers as postmodern fragmented selves and consumers as seekers of a coherent sense of self' (Patterson and Schroeder 2010, p. 253).

The most dominant discourse in tattoo narrative has been the expression of personal growth. This narrative connects with empowerment, spiritual growth and overcoming adversity or trauma (Sarnecki 2001; Park and Helgeson 2006). The appraised meaning of the life-changing event is assimilated and forms part of the understanding of the identity narrative. It can represent *freedom from* or *overcoming* life events, or just celebrating and decorating the beauty of the body (Fisher 2002). The narrative of memorial tattoos has seen a massive rise over the last ten years. This is partly encouraged by the media and the growing number of television programmes dedicated to tattoos. It has also created a surge in tattoo-based research, particularly in America (e.g. Alcina 2009; Samuel 2011; Anastasia 2009; Littell 2003).

Gergen (1995) and Polkinghorne (2001) argue for a reconceptualization of the traditional Maslow and Rogerian theories of self to include wider humanistic views and beliefs (McDonald and Wearing 2013). Not that Polkinghorne considered the actualization tendency theory to be inaccurate, but just lacking the sociocultural influence on self. These researchers advocated Heidegger and Foucault's view of the self as being constituted by its social and cultural conditions (McDonald and Wearing 2013). With Rogers (1961), viewing the self in terms of *actual self* (untouched by external influence*)* and *self-concept* (how each person views themselves*)*, I feel these self-theories fail to address what Geller termed, the *true self* (Geller 1982). This is our genetic predisposition to adapt to cultural influences. If we are all born the same – *untouched* – we all have the ability to adapt into the culture into which we are born, and the flexibility to change. Social and cultural impact is therefore unavoidable when exploring selfhood. And as we express our phenomenological sense of who we are to our conscious mind (Horrocks and Jevtic 1997), we do it in a socially constructed way. To this, Rogers would argue that it is within these modern and culturally defined constructions that we distort and lose sight of our *authentic self* (Rogers 1961). The *real self* is 'something which is comfortably discovered in one's own experiences, not something imposed upon' (Rogers 1961, p. 114).

Identity narratives flow out of our sense of who we are and how we experience ourselves in everyday life. Without an interpretive stance or a context in which we exist, there is no consciousness (Smith et al. 2009) to our experience of who we are and this in turn *cuts off* our identity narrative, sense of self and tattoo narrative. If our identity narrative is informed by our sense of self, a tattoo would be a visual presentation of that sense of self. And as we are in constant flow (Rogers 1961), we have the opportunity to rewrite our identity narrative all the time. Alcina (2009) would argue that identity is anchored through continuous narrative and that the tattoo is the anchor. According to Giddens (1991), discovering our authentic self is a process of shedding false self, or former beliefs, to uncover true self. The identity of the self is an ongoing routine, sustained by reflexive and conscious awareness (Giddens 1991). Kosut contends how tattoos are a visual reminder of these parts of self. They are current or previous presentations of ourselves that 'ground our story on the body' (Kosut 2000, p. 90). This research highlights a magnitude of statements of tattoo wearers that spoke of each tattoo representing 'a part of me', or a 'particular time in my life' (Kosut 2000; Lemma 2010; Zimmer 2011; DeMello 2000, Albin 2006). To Giddens (1991), the existential question of self-identity depends on how long a person can keep the particular narrative going. When thinking about the permanence of tattoos, it can appear that tattoos are the way of keeping a particular narrative permanent and ongoing.

> As long as we remain preoccupied with questions of identity, we will continue to manipulate our bodies and to 'customise' them to lend form and meaning to our personal and social identities. Body modification marks

the body, inscribes it, and so constructs it within physical, cultural and even political fields (Lemma 2010, p. 15).

Wittgenstein reminds us of the relation between the Body and Self (Giddens 1991). The Self is embodied and creates an organic process of thought, meaning-making and language (Johnson 2007). Although the Body is an object in which we dwell, it isn't just a mechanical entity that gets us from A to B. It is through corporeal immersion of everyday interactions with others and our daily tasks that help maintain our sense of self. In a postmodern culture, Shilling explains how the body has become a 'body project' – space for self-expression and transformation. This concept explicates the Western view that the body is a project that needs to be 'worked out and accomplished as part of an individual's self-identity' in order to make any meaning (Shilling 1993). This identity reconstruction has in itself become a challenge (Klesse 2000), but one that has been met by a consumer culture that has provided a marketplace with an array of 'symbolic resources' and merchandise in the maintenance of self-identity and narrative (Patterson and Schroeder 2010, p. 254). Giddens (1991) would contend this drive to identify in our consumer culture, as driven by our detachment from our traditional systems of meaning, forcing us into a state of constant reflexivity and search for present meaning and identity. This puts us in a permanent cycle of identity re-shifting, with the body as the axis. Erik Erikson (1993) spoke of how our traditions and customs served as anchors for a secure Sense of Self and sense of belonging – something that has been lost in this modern age of consumer culture.

In the meantime, the body project will continue until a point of accomplishment is reached. With the focus of tattoos as body projects, Pitts discusses fresh tattoo aftercare.

Meaning is attached to the feeling of accomplishment in coping with the pain of receiving a tattoo. This is followed by tending to a healing scar. Previous research suggests this to be quite a significant process, especially among post-trauma memorial tattoos (Caruth 1996). This can be quite a reflexive process, participating in self-care and self-attention (Pitts, 2003) until the scar has healed, similar perhaps to the original injury. This reinforces Caruth's idea that 'we are compelled to repeat the trauma in some new, creative setting that will allow for a different, life affirming signification of the event while still bearing witness to it'. (Sarnecki 2001, p. 37). The body project is completed when a feeling of embodiedness is reached.

From a qualitative perspective, this 'feeling' of completion and the emotion attached to it is in a sense how we experience meaning. It has been notoriously hard to analyse and theorize this subjective stance as philosophers would describe feelings as 'non-cognitive' and as having no role in *meaning*. Heidegger contended that the quality of being human has been neglected in research, either because it was taken for granted or because the understanding of Dasein was inaccessible (Smith et al. 2009). The focus of most theories of meaning and qualitative experience lies with conceptual-propositional skeletal structures of meaning (Johnson 2007; Bonanno and Keltner 2004; Neimeyer 2001). However, phenomenology does not bypass emotion, feelings and *quality* in meaning-making (Smith and Osborn 1998; Johnson 2007). Johnson argues that we cannot 'capture qualitative experience in propositions with subject-predicate structure; we tend to downplay the importance of qualities as part of meaning' (Johnson 2007, p. 70). The whole beauty of qualitative experiencing of things and objects is what gives personal meaning to them. The meaning we take from things or events depends on our experiencing, and on assessing the qualities of that lived-experience, e.g. the smell that meets me when I open my front door tells me I am home at a more profound level than intellectually knowing I'm at home. There are no words involved in this exercise, just pure subjective connection with what is being experienced and the meaning I take from everyday experience. In *Tricks of Time,* Muldoon (2006) discusses Merleau-Ponty's stance that there is no adequate way to capture the essence of 'being–in-the-world' (p. 160), rendering the meaning-making process as uncertain which has led the cognitivist approach to argue that meaning can only be created through the use of language (White 2007). 'It is the structure of narrative that provides the principal frame of intelligibility for acts of meaning-making' (White 2007, p. 80). Johnson counteracts this argument by exploring personal meaning one can take from staring at a painting or watching a piece of interpretive dance. There are no words involved with this exercise, yet the person would have had a subjective connection and an opportunity to create personal meaning (Johnson 2007). In this research of tattoos, personal meaning can be incorporated into Johnson's idea of embodied meaning and art. Participants discussed their individual experiences of meaning in tattoo design/image, meaning behind the permanence of a tattoo, meaning to their identity formation and how meaning can shift and change.

Participants

As my area of interest was very specific, I recruited a purposive (non-probability) sampling of four tattooed Counsellors. My inclusion criteria were: qualified Counsellors or Counsellors in training (excluding first year students) of any training background, who have tattoos with significant personal meaning. My rationale for choosing this sample was due to Counsellors' levels of self-awareness and personal development reached and the existence of psychological support, although participants were inter-viewed as 'people' rather than Counsellors. I assigned each participant with a code name to protect their identity. I included both men and women (see Table 1 for details of the participants).

Participant	JB	ST	BF	FC
Gender	Male	Female	Female	Female
Age range	30–39	40–49	50–59	50–59
Training	Integrative	Sex Therapist	Integrative	Psychodynamic

Table 1. Details of participants.

Data collection

I found the method of semi-structured interviews of data collection most compatible with qualitative research and methods of analysis. The questions asked were:

- Did your tattoo represent anything special to you at the time you got it?
- Has that meaning changed at all?
- Why did you choose that specific design?
- Why did you choose to have a tattoo specifically?
- What do people around you think of it?
- Do you, or would you, have any more?

Interviews were arranged at the various offices and college facilities of the participants. All rooms complied with con-fidentiality and recording needs. All interviews were digitally recorded for transcription. All participants signed the consent form for audio recording.

Findings

Three master themes emerged with subsequent sub-themes:

Master themes	1 - Self	2 - Tattoo Narrative	3 - Meaning-making of Tattoo Narrative
Sub-themes		2.1 Spiritual	3.1 Permanence
		2.2 Personal growth	3.2 Location
		2.3 Memorial/tribute	3.3 Design
		2.4 Individualism/ Collectivism	3.4 Utility

Table 2. Emerging themes.

Master theme 1: Self

The master theme, Self, produced no sub-themes. All four participants, however, reflected on their Sense of Self throughout the interviews in a variety of ways, all resulting in a type of 'I am the type of person who ...' statements. Participants reflected on who they used to be, their changing identities and who they are at this point in their lives. This master theme captured all those 'I' statements that related to the person they are, rather than their tattoo.

ST explains the Self she was when she received this particular tattoo. "*I was married for 15 years, single for 9 years, and when I had this tattoo, I was probably single for 4 years ... and I was mental. Absolutely mental ... But I think, back then there was massively two sides to me ... I have absolutely no issue about anybody knowing anything. I'm really, really ridiculously open*" (ST). BF explored the Self she was, the breaking of that mould of conditions of worth and the Self she since became: "*I never put a foot out ... I was a pleaser ... I was always trying to earn my mother's love, and I still haven't got it ... there is something about that word 'offensive' ... no one's gonna like me, because it's offensive. I was then starting to probably have a voice. I've done it once, it didn't particularly hurt, I got through it ... Uhm ... I can do it again. No-one rejected me for it. I'm not a bad person for it ..."* (BF). FC explored her spiritual Self and how her years of meditation, Reiki practice and Personal Development (PD) have created the energy flow that she feels in her every day: *"I have looked in very great depth into who I am, who am I ... I am still getting to know myself ... not myself as a Frances but my spiritual self, my real, my true self, not the ego, or the mannerisms or the personality, but the spirit of me ... in the letting go that I found I'm opening up more, ... but the more I let go, the more I'm able to open up to the spirituality all around me and within me, and the whole and the one and the 'Om' and other people as the spirit in them. I still find it difficult to communicate my ideas and my thoughts to others. I feel that everything else seems to be in place, but I do need to do some work on my throat chakra"* (FC). JB spoke passionately of the powerful feeling a tattoo gave him in claiming his changing identity: *"'Yeah, I'm tattooed', I felt cool, I didn't feel blank. I was gaining a part of my identity, or I realized that I was... but to make a statement on my body about who I really was ... wow! That really was powerful, because it was me and this is a mirror now and I can look at my tattoo and I know who I am ... uhm ... I'm making a statement about when I changed as a person, or when I achieved something or when I overcame a challenge ..."* (JB). The findings suggest the significant role reflexivity, personal history and individual memory play in understanding participants' sense of Self.

Master theme 2: Tattoo Narrative:
This master theme of 'Tattoo Narrative' produced four sub-themes and reflects most of the type of narratives discussed in tattoo narrative literature.

Sub-theme 2.1: Spiritual: FC's tattoo narrative demonstrates the level of personal and spiritual meaning her tattoo carries: *"... when you go into meditation and then you get the silence ... it's like beneath the silence ..., it's like a part of the silence. A part of the silence is ... it is the silence. I couldn't even voice it, because it seems like it's a ... it's like ... the earth, it's like the sound of the earth, the sound of the universe. And to me ... I wanna be part of that and to be part of that ... like it has given me a feeling of being a part of the whole, the one, the om, the universe, God, Spirit, whatever. I feel like this tattoo has imprinted itself in on me ... it's part of me, so I feel part of the one now ..."* (FC).

Sub-theme 2.2: Personal growth: ST discussed three different tattoos. One of the three tattoos she discussed reflects her personal growth tattoo narrative. It's a tattoo she received to mark the end of a long developmental journey: *"... so I wanted the word 'Sex' in Greek and this was just at the end of my postgraduate ... and I was about to graduate and I was so proud of myself, because I've been through hell and high water to get where I wanted to be, and I was so pleased with meself"* (ST).

Sub-theme 2.3: Memorial/tribute: This sub-theme represents tattoos that are a memorial to a deceased loved one, but also tributes of love to people that are still alive. Two of the four participants reflected this tattoo narrative. JB talks about how his tattoo and future tattoos will mark the chapters of his life – acting as if a tribute to his life. His tattoo is a tribute to the relationship he has with his son. *"I remember what it meant to me then and wow it was cool what happened from this tattoo to this tattoo, these things have happened in my life, and these things are the headings, the chapters of how I have experienced life ... and it meant a lot to get a tattoo for me, because it was about that relationship with my son"* (JB). BF's tattoo narrative for one of her tattoos pays homage to her departed father: *"My father was – he loved his gardening – and there was this buddleia tree and* *it was always butterflies. So for that, it's me and him … it's from the father through having my children to where I am now with my partner … yeah … to where I am today. Yeah … that I love dearly"* (BF).

Sub-theme 2.4: Individual/collectivism: ST expressed her fundamental narrative as being an expression of how similar and also how different she is to her fellow man: *"… and that's why I wanted this tattoo, because I'm saying to everybody out there that I am actually fundamentally just like you, but them two little strands at the bottom say … 'but I'm made differently, ultimately as I grow up in what I learn and what I do.' So from being 14, I've been six foot, so I was Big Bird, and then it got shortened to Bird and everybody calls me Bird"* (ST). JB highlighted a feeling of connection with fellow tattooed individuals: *"From a comment or question about something on your body, all of a sudden you're building a relationship with people who you never would speak to. And then you could find common values, like being a good parent … to get people who I wouldn't normally talk to, to open myself up conversationally and I can talk about theirs, you know? Lots of new beginnings… What should we talk about? All of a sudden you're – bang (click of the fingers) – you're straight into who they really are, and who you really are"* (JB). It is evident from these findings that all participants connected to a specific tattoo narrative. The following master theme explains the meaning participants connect to their tattoos.

Master theme 3: Meaning-making of Tattoo Narratives

This master theme captured four elements of meaning-making for the participants: Permanence, meaning in location, meaning in design, and the tattoo's utility:

Sub-theme 3.1: Permanence: Each participant spoke about the meaning of *permanence* of their tattoos. What was interesting is how each statement related to their tattoo narrative. JB's tattoo narrative of memorial/tribute suggests replacing the loss of the family unit, with a reminder that his son will permanently be his: *"I'm thinking maybe there was a part of me that had to keep something alive from that relationship, but that's just a small part ... this tattoo on my arm has only made up in a small part of the relationship with her, it's more about him"* (JB). BF's tattoo narrative highlights the replacement of a loss with permanence – the loss of her father. *"That's it ... they're mine. No-one can take them away from me. Yeah ... they're permanent. As I'm just sitting here, I'm now thinking of my dad dying, ... something's been taken away from me, uhmm ... my mother not loving me"* (BF). ST introduced a conflict to the permanence element of tattoos. When talking about the individual/collectivism element of her DNA strand tattoo, she stated, *"... But the tattoo was just something I wanted permanently symbolizing it ..."* (ST). When discussing regret of a specific tattoo's location, she stated, *"... you can do anything like that nowadays, it's not a problem. ... you wanna move something, move. You wanna ... you know like ... awww you have a tattoo you got it for life. That's not the case anymore"* (ST). FC reflected on the permanence of her spirituality and how her chosen tattoo reflected that point: *"that is* (the tattoo) *like a sign for me to say 'This is permanent, this is who I am. I'm a spiritual person, take it or leave it. This, this, this is me... because it's permanent and I believe in it so much that I will put it on my body, for ever. I love my tattoo, I absolutely love it'"* (FC). Following a discussion with another person about her choice of *"being 'marked for life'"* she said, *"I'm not covered in scars, I'm not marked for life with scars – I like it! ... I chose this one. The others were accidents"* (FC).

Sub-theme 3.2: Location: All four participants connected meaning with the location of their tattoos. *"I play orthodox grip, so my forearm is facing me and I'm playing for my son cos it faces me when I'm playing"* [JB], *"… the butterfly is, for me, particularly larger, the largest one. And … it is hidden from me, but I think I'm the most uncomfortable about it, because of its size"* [BF]. ST spoke of how important *location choice* can be in the case of regret of getting her hand tattooed. The last *in vivo* quote is about a different tattoo where the location was important to her. At this stage of her life, she strongly identified with a character from a television series and had the same tattoo of the character tattooed on her shoulder: *"And me dad said to me 'You shouldn't 've had it on your hand'… and that bothers me, because me dad … it's only me and me dad … but I just thought … because I had doubts and when he said that, I thought 'Oh he's right'. I was so excited … and I was like 'oh no no no, I wanna be proud when people ask what it is', and, you know, this and that and the other. So I'm having it removed to have it done behind my ear now, cos I listen to sex all the time. So it's about listening to sex … And I just thought 'Oh God', and I just thought I've made a mistake … one of the reasons why I had this on my shoulder at the time, … that was the meaning behind it. But one of the characters in the show has the tattoo on her shoulder in exactly the same place"* (ST). Even though the location for FC was very important to the meaning of her tattoo, she did find herself questioning whether this was the real reason behind her location choice: *"My intention is to get a tattoo on every chakra point. … I've often questioned myself, why didn't you get it done on your arm, or … Why have you got it hidden – for something that is so important … I could be in denial!! … I'm in denial of wanting to hide it because I'm not confident enough to … maybe to show it, but it doesn't feel like that. It feels like I don't want to just put it out there"* (FC).

Sub-theme 3.3: Design: Each participant connected great personal meaning to each tattoo. BF spoke of how her mother never even knew what her favourite colour was as a child. This was something she consciously chose to mark in all her tattoos. *"… it would always be the blue option … but I didn't like blue! I actually liked green …"* (BF). JB commemorated the personal meaning and history Thailand had for him, by choosing to have his son's name tattooed in Thai lettering. *"… this idea of writing (I did English Lit at Uni) and words, names … for me that's where the meaning is. I could have had an illustration or something symbolic, but I just wanted his name … I thought this place has meaning for me. It's where I go to get away from the world for a bit. To sit on a desert island and just stare into space. So that connection with a part of myself … uhm … to get it done in Thai …"* (JB). ST is fascinated by the Nature/Nurture debate and the influence of genetics on our DNA. At the same time as her research into the topic, she started watching a television programme that incorporated this debate with *"the uniqueness of us"*. Her tattoo is from this particular television programme: *"… the people who knew the programme and knew what it meant … they'd come up and they'd go … 'Oh my god, a helix … you've got a helix! … How cool is she, she's got a helix of Heroes on her shoulder'"* (ST). FC's tattoo is the symbol of universal sound and having this powerful symbol imprinted on her body feels like she can draw from its energy. *"I feel like this tattoo has imprinted itself in on me, so that symbol has the power of … it has its own power being with me. It has – because the symbol itself is a powerful symbol – I believe that that powerful symbol is part of me now"* (FC).

Sub-theme 3.4: Utility: It is my understanding from listening to my participants, that tattoos with significant meaning also have a purpose. ST used her DNA helix tattoo to illustrate this point: *"… it just <u>reminds</u> me, I own it, that I'm no better than anybody else"* (ST). FC's tattoo has made her question its message to her: *"It's a part of me, but it does not seem to make sense that the particular tattoo I've got at the moment is the universal sound. Perhaps to me that is the sound that I need, this is* *the universal sound that perhaps I need to be heard, perhaps I need to show myself that ... I do need a <u>reminder</u> now and again. Perhaps I do, when I'm getting angry or stroppy with the family, or not being as nice as I could be"* (FC). BF's tattoo journey reflects how she has developed and changed over her lifespan and reflects the freedom she now feels: *"Freedom to choose, freedom to have an opinion ... and it doesn't matter what other people think of them ... Yeah. ... it's a reminder ... It's my life really. So, it's from the father through having my children to where I am now with my partner ... yeah ... to where I am today. Yeah ... that I love dearly"* (BF). JB explored how his tattoo serves as a statement to himself and his son, *"... it was about me making a statement, that's what it is, a visual statement ... uhm ... of my intentions about being a good dad ... I'm looking at it every day ... I'm <u>reminded</u> every day and it ... it did what it was supposed to do. I came to realize that it is also a <u>reminder</u> to me to support my dreams, because in order to be the kind of dad that I want to be. There's something that I have to fulfil within me ... that he can look back on. So it's just as much a <u>reminder</u> to me, about my goals and my dreams and my values, as it is about him"* (JB). The significant findings from this master theme show that meaning can be found in all elements of tattoos – from design, to location. Meaning is connected to the permanence of the image and serves a meaningful purpose.

Discussion

I use the term Phenomenological Sense of Self to situate this research in relation to self-theory. I find it important to highlight the delicate process of discussing self-theory without reference to a theoretical understanding of the self. This is because Phenomenology is the suspended view of how I experienced the participant's sense of self and it is NOT about my understanding of a particular behaviouristic theory per se. Saying that, I am not a blank sheet and it is inevitable that I bring with me, my own beliefs, values and assumptions. Finlay calls this, 'something of a dance – the researcher slides between striving for reductive focus and reflexive self-awareness; between bracketing pre-understandings and exploiting them as a source of insight' (Finlay 2008, p. 1). Keeping the dance going, I was also conscious of how no two individual's lived-experiences are the same. With this in mind, I found it important to treat each participant's sense of self as the individuals they are and didn't think sub-themes would be appropriate to the master theme, Self.

Participants have, however, discussed a range of topics related to their sense of self. My sense-making of this related to counselling theory in the form of configurations of self, a changing self and personal development of self. As my participants and I are all Counsellors, it felt acceptable for me to grab on to counselling theory as an anchor, until I came to a point of understanding the engagement of bracketing and exploiting theory as a source of insight. The majority of participants discussed their sense of self through sharing their configurations of self, their true/authentic self and how some have shed conditions of worth. A key point I've found is that all participants reflected a sense of ongoing change and development. This finding concurs with Giddens's view that discovering our authentic self is a process of shedding false self or former beliefs. The identity of the self is an ongoing routine, sustained by reflexive and conscious awareness (Giddens 1991). This was the case for all participants. However, as each person's lived-experience is so subjective, I didn't want to generalize on every aspect of my findings and lose the essence of each participant. With this in mind, the following few paragraphs will reflect my interpretative discussion on the individual transcript findings.

ST described her self-concept as being ridiculously open, not caring what others knew or thought of her. To her, she had very distinguishable sides – *"an angel side"* and a *"devil side"*, she had a *"medical head"* and a *"psychological head"*, she used to be married, and then single for four years, she was *"mental"*. Some of these configurations explain the person she is, but also versions of former selves. As Mearns and Thorne contend, 'configurations of the self are available to the individual that emerge at different times to take into account the differing circumstances that an individual confronts in life' (Mearns and Thorne 2000, p. 107). These versions of self (and at different times in ST's life) have been reflected through her tattoos and identity narrative.

As mentioned previously, my findings suggest that the self is not a fixed structure, but can shed the 'conditioned self' to become her true self (Merry 2002). Through BF's personal development towards becoming a Counsellor, it became evident how tied she used to be in her conditions of worth. She *"was a pleaser*, she *never put a foot wrong"*, she was *"always trying to earn her mother's love"*. She used the idiom, *"breaking the mould"* to articulate just how ingrained her conditioned self was and the process by which she started on the road to self-discovery. When we shed our conditions of worth, we start to trust our internal locus of evaluation, our trustworthy organism (Rogers 1961). BF started with body modification in the form of piercings and discovered that *"no one rejected her for it"*. Others' approval or disapproval didn't matter anymore. To BF, she *"was starting to find her voice"*. In Rogerian terms, she was striving to become a fully functioning person, shedding her external locus of evaluation and focused inwards towards her need to actualize her conditioned self (Rogers 1961).

Part of being a Counsellor involves a high level of commitment to personal development. Some participants spoke of finding or recovering their true self. According to Rogers, this is the authentic self that gets distorted by culturally defined constructions we live with in the modern day. FC described a beautiful moment of this journey to self-discovery. She has discovered that *"the more I let go, the more I'm able to open up to the spirituality all around me and within me, and the whole and the one and the 'Om' and other people as the spirit in them"* (FC). In existential terms, she meets others at relational depth (Mearns and Thorne 2000). FC recognizes her spiritual self and trusts her organismic self to open up (as opposed to staying closed-off) and surrender to the spiritual experience of meditation and connecting with others. There is another element to FC's view of what her self is capable and not capable of at present. Personal development and self-awareness is so intrinsic with her present personal journey, that she has become aware of her difficulty to communicate her own needs and thoughts. She is open to co-experience the journey of others (as a Counsellor) and to experience a connection with those around her, but needs to do work on why she is finding it so hard to express her own needs. This just reflects the fluid and ongoing nature of the self and the innate striving to self-actualize. Rogers calls this the experience of comfortably discovering the real self (Rogers 1961). This discovering was also evident in the discourse of JB. My interpretation of the text related to self, illuminated a young man who suffered the trauma of a severed attachment with his own father. JB mentioned what got him through that particular event, was the thought of how he would be a different dad to what his father was. This painful memory played such a pivotal part in JB's development of self and his tattoo (his *mirror*) reminds him NOT to be like his own father.

Furthermore, reflexive thoughts around what it meant to gain and incorporate this new part of his identity show how powerful this statement was to him and his confidence. He has shed some of his father's values and used the resilience he gained from the experience, as a life lesson.

> Tattoo stories centralize one experience – the tattoo – and relate what changes have occurred in that tattoo wearer's life since that central defining point. Tattoo narratives, however, are different from other types of life-story narratives in that they do not rely so heavily on memory and are much more self-reflexive (DeMello 2000, p. 152).

As mentioned earlier, identity narratives flow out of our sense of who we are and how we experience ourselves in everyday life. Heidegger viewed the self as a human construction, a way of being in the world. Without an interpretive stance or a context in which we exist, there is no consciousness (Smith et al. 2009) to our experience of who we are and this in turn *cuts off* our identity narrative, sense of self and tattoo narrative. My findings show that all participants related to a particular tattoo narrative, but again, each narrative was different from the other. I therefore cannot generalize across my findings.

FC's entire interview was based in the discourse of Spirituality. Previous studies on how language has been used to illustrate the phenomenological connection with Spirituality are in abundance (Gockel 2009; Bruner 1990). Schwab and Frances (2013) and Riessman (2000) highlighted a variety of meaning-making strategies people use to make sense of their spiritually based story narratives. With this current research I am highlighting the spirituality narrative in a slightly different way – by means of a tattoo narrative. FC's tattoo makes her feel connected to *"part of the whole, the one, the om, the universe, God, Spirit"*. Being deeply connected to the earth and spirit and feeling as if she is part of that energy flow, is what her tattoo represents for her. Tattoo-based research found the experience of being tattooed as spiritualistic or ritualistic (Goode and Vail 2008). Not used as an excerpt in my findings, but quite relevant to this section, was FC's lived-experience of receiving her tattoo. She described the experience as *"not making sense, but I liked the feeling of getting it done"*. She reflected on the connection she felt to the music that was playing in the background and how the heavy metal song represented *"the idea of how a tattoo feels through sound"*. My interpretation of her account also felt spiritual, like a deeper connection through penetration of the tattoo needle, reflecting similar experiences mentioned by the Modern Primitive tattoo community (Klesse 2000).

The most dominant tattoo narrative in research has been the narrative of personal growth through self-help and empowerment (DeMello 2000; Fisher 2002). Sarneki offered the view that tattooing could be a mark of the 'ability to control or master stressful events' when a person could feel out of control (Sarneki 2001, p. 21). Often, people in stressful life situations would reach 'turning points' that fundamentally change the person's current life course, leading to personal growth, overcoming a trauma and a changing identity (Riessman 2000). In this research, the majority of participants mentioned their own growth, change and development, but only ST chose to commemorate this aspect of her challenging journey with a tattoo. She described the experience of training as a Sex Therapist, as going *"through hell and high water"*. She held on to an image of the word 'Sex' in Greek for ten years before she qualified and finally had it tattooed on her body. She needed to complete this journey of going to hell and back first. The tattoo was her mark of completion. She was now a Sex Therapist and could allow herself to have it marked on her skin.

The connection between memorial tattoos and mourning has been highly researched over the last ten years (Alcina 2009; Samuel 2011; Anastasia 2009; Littell 2003). I believe this has been as a result of a cultural shift and an embracing of tattoos through popular culture and media. It was through the volume of tattoo-based television programmes that I became interested in the area. There is something so moving in re-creating a continuing bond with a deceased loved one through a memorial tattoo. BF recalled playing with her father in the garden as a child. There were always butterflies around the buddleia tree. It was just her and her dad. The attachment to him was secure, unlike her mother. She lost her dad when she was aged six. In order to protect herself, she had the tattoo placed on her back where she cannot see it every day, but she knows it is there. As mentioned previously, this statement suggests that not all memorial tattoo wearers wish to see their tattoo on a daily basis, as previous research might have found. I chose to use the word, Tribute as a narrative to describe a tattoo that represents a loved one that is still alive. JB explained how, one day, he wants to look back at his tattoos, reading them like chapters to the significant events in his life. The birth of his son, marked the first chapter. This is a tattoo that JB is proud of, *"... yes, I am tattooed. I am not blank any more"* and *"I can look at my tattoo and I know who I am"* are very powerful statements of his tattooed identity.

The literature on tattoo narratives suggests that one way to express individuality is through a custom tattoo (DeMello 2000). So if we were just to engage with ST's DNA helix that she copied from the television show, it wouldn't appear to be individual at all. To me, this is where reflexivity, connection and personal meaning steps in. ST didn't choose this image because she wanted a tattoo that made a statement about her individuality in tattoo choice. ST chose this tattoo to highlight her sameness, but also her differences as a human being. For her, she belongs to a community of biological human beings. This suggests that perhaps she sees it as a source of identification to the human race, and not just as a source to identify to a tattoo community as Moerier et al. (2011) would argue. For one participant, however, this identification to a tattoo community was a revelation. Since receiving his tattoo on his forearm, JB experienced a feeling of connection with fellow tattooed people. He was astonished how new relationships seemed to form in his life. Through sharing his tattoo narrative, an instant connection with the core value of another human being was created. My interpretation, while reflexively restraining my pre-understandings of this phenomenon, conjures up the idea of being part of a community. As Anderson (1983) re-defined community as no longer 'village-based' (Anderson 1983, cited in DeMello 2000) or concrete. Today's communities are more imagined and 'must be understood with respect to the style in which they are imagined, i.e., via shared ties of kinship, citizenship … Communities like the tattoo community provide a model for just such an understanding, in that they do not even possess the quality of spatial boundedness that nations, cities, or neighbourhoods have' (DeMello 2000, p. 40). Because of this imagined and non-concreted form of new community, members need to seek out other members in order to form connections and a shared identity. What makes the tattoo community different from more traditional communities, like occupation or religion, is its emphasis on individual choice in the expression of self-identity (DeMello 2000). Muggleton (1995) noted a movement towards 'neo-tribalism' with a strong emphasis on personal nature of modification rather than subculture affiliation of more traditional and class-fixed tattoos like gang affiliates. Patterson and Schroeder explored embodied identity within consumer research and generated a series of insights into intercorporeality, embodiment and body projects. They challenged the idea that we are relatively self-contained and solely responsible for our own identity construction. Their findings suggest that our identities are socially constructed and understood through 'the works, looks and discourses of others' (Patterson and Schroeder 2010, p. 263).

> Engaging this attitude involves a preparedness to be open to whatever may emerge rather than prejudging or prestructuring one's findings. The aim is to connect directly and immediately with the world as we (and, through empathy, as our research participants) experience it (Finlay 2008, p. 4).

An element that has emerged from this research that I wasn't anticipating was the meaning the participants attached to the permanence of a tattoo. There has been a clear link between each tattoo narrative and permanence, regardless of type of tattoo narrative. Previous research has highlighted the importance that some individuals place on replacing a loss with something that cannot be lost (Follett 2009). The permanence of tattoos has given some participants this opportunity as can be seen in the account of BF and the memorial butterfly tattoo she had done in the name of her deceased father. There is a drive or a need for something to continue beyond the loss (Follett 2009). A tattoo can create this continuing bond. It is the one thing no one can take away, and the meaning of this has proven to be immensely powerful in all the participants' narratives. ST wanted her belief system of individuality in a collectivist world permanently symbolized. FC wanted the permanence of her spirituality forever reflected on her embodied self. During the interview with FC, she mentioned her husband's disapproval of her tattoo, stating that she is 'marked for life now'. Her reply to this was that she chose this mark and that all her other marks were scars from accidents. This carried great importance to her – her permanent reflection of her true self, not a disfigurement that life threw at her in a form of an accidental scar.

The chosen location of the tattoo in itself can hold meaning for the tattooed. It was interesting that each participant brought the topic of location, but in completely different ways. Fisher wrote,

> Having this decorative function, tattoos are often associated with exhibitionism. Although there is indeed an element of desire to reveal tattoos, there is often an equally profound desire to conceal tattoos. Revealing the tattoo has several functions, including showing the individual's stylishness, identifying a group to which they belong, and demonstrating their rebelliousness. The desire to conceal can stem from the deeply personal meaning of the tattoo for the individual or from the deeply embedded social stigma. While the tattooed person enjoys the positive attention from his/her peers generated by the tattoo, most of these same people feel embarrassed about the negative reactions they get from others, especially when this reaction is coming from friends and family. People with tattoos try to avoid and resent questions such as 'Why would you do that to yourself?' (Fisher 2002, p. 12).

To JB, it was important to have his son's name on his forearm, visible when he plays the drums, reminding him to follow his own dreams, but also as a reminder to encourage his son to do the same one day. FC reflected an element of Fisher's (2002) findings. Although her initial thought behind her tattoo location was so strongly connected to her chakra points, she did question whether her concealed tattoo location reflected her lack of confidence as she didn't have it more on show. This was a very reflexive moment for her during the interview and she came to the conclusion that she *"doesn't want to put it just out there"*. BF admitted to feeling uncomfortable with the size of her memorial tattoo and explored the idea why she chose this particular tattoo to go on her back so that she doesn't see it every day. ST discussed the tattoo location of two different tattoos. The first location was purely due to identification with a television character that had the same tattoo on her shoulder. The second tattoo brought a new element to permanence. ST regretted a specific tattoo location. This brought a new dimension to tattoo research, as all available research discussed the regret of a tattoo and not just tattoo location (Follett 2009; Sanders and Vail 2008; Armstrong 1994; Atkinson 2004). This participant is in the process of having the tattoo removed and then re-done in a different and more significant location – behind her ear, as she is a Sex Therapist and she listens to *"sex all the time"*. From having the tattoo on her hand, she was bombarded with people wanting to know the meaning of it. ST would describe herself as a *"ridiculously open person"*, but she still found it an intrusion when she just wanted to get on with her shopping. This 'moving' of the tattoo has also brought up the debate of how permanent a tattoo really has to be in the modern days of laser removal. Follett (2009) highlights the scarification and that in itself will stay permanent, but immersing myself in ST's discourse, I didn't get a sense that this was an issue to her.

It feels a bit obvious to discuss the importance of design to a permanent image, but what is interesting is the level of detail of meaning-making that is put into the design that is then reflected in what a person has tattooed on them, even to the extent of the colours they choose to include. All BF's tattoos are a shade of green. This has been a very deliberate statement for her. She reflected on how she always loved green, but that her mother never even knew this. Her mother discarded her preference and always dressed her in blue. By having her tattoos in green, she claims her favourite colour. The meaning that she has taken from this, reflects her assessment of that lived-experience, of being a child and not being able to express herself (Johnson 2007). For JB, it was clear that he wanted his son's name represented with lettering and not an image. Words are where this participant attaches meaning. As a child, he received the value from his father that names are more important than images. He grew up to study English Literature because to him, a word is what carries meaning. He chose to have his son's name written in Thai lettering, as this reflected the emotional and meaningful connection he wanted to hold on to with Thailand. This is the place he can escape to, where he can *"connect with a part of himself"*. This is where he went after his marriage dissolved, where he came to take stock and to have his son's name immortalized on his arm. It would imply that the meaning this participant takes from his tattoo design is that it keeps him connected to the history and time he spent with his ex-wife in Thailand, and the boy that was created through that significant timeframe. Also, that the use of language might have been a condition of worth or value passed on from his own father (Merry 2002).

What has been illuminated during this research has been the understanding that tattoos with significant meaning also serve a purpose. These tattoos serve as a poignant reminder to each person's personal life message (Pitts 2003). Alcina calls these, 'note-to-self tattoos' (Alcina 2009, p. 64). She categorized reminders under three headings: 'important people, important places and tattoos as symbolic of a life philosophy by which they are trying to live or character traits to which they aspire' (Alcina 2009, p. 65). My interpretation matches that of Alcina. For ST, it is a reminder that she is *"no better than anybody else"*. To FC, it is a reminder to not get so angry and to stay in the calm and peaceful space that she enters when she meditates. It is also a reminder to her to *"show herself more"* and that she too has to *"be heard"*. During BF's journey of self-discovery and change, her tattoos remind her of the freedom she discovered she had, once she shed the shackles of her conditions of worth. It is also a reminder of the things in life that she loves dearly. To JB, it is a reminder to not just follow his own dreams, but to guide his son to do the same.

Conclusion

IPA is limited to small-scale or time-limited studies. The methods are not appropriate for larger number of 'faceless' participants. It is in the nature of IPA to explore and seek out individual phenomenology. As participation was self-selected, it did not represent a cross-section of the population. Although I had both male and female Counsellor participants, all four were from the same ethnicity (i.e. white). As this is a small-scale, qualitative study, findings cannot be generalized.

However, conducting this research has given me a front row seat in the delicate process of individual meaning-making and understanding the self in its lived world. Through the immortalization of words or an image on a person's body, I gained an understanding of phenomeno-logical accounts of personal growth and identification. Also of integrating versions of self, previous and present. As a researcher, I witnessed their 'embodied visual communi-cation' – permanent messages or reminders of that particular self they were when they received this tattoo (Kosut 2000, p. 98). The research highlighted the importance of the utility of the tattoo. I have always considered tattoo narratives as such poignant forms of sharing phenomenological selfhood. Listening to people's accounts from all walks of life always made me think of a missed opportunity in the counselling room. I often found myself wondering whether non-tattooed Counsellors ever considered asking a tattooed client about their tattoos. In my experience, it can be such an illuminating aid.

CHAPTER TWO

THE IMPACT OF PERSON-CENTRED COUNSELLING TRAINING ON FRIENDSHIP

Kathryn Hackland

Introduction

This study has grown out of my experiences of friendship, whilst training to be a Person-Centred Counsellor. For me, there has been a maturing process of self-discovery that has not only illuminated my own 'workings' within my family bonds, but also in my social relationships as I notice, and re-position myself, 'within' my friendships. Existing work notes how the 'clandestine activity' (Egan 1973) and 'emotional separateness' (Lerner 1989, p. 212) of both the work and personal development of the therapist, can really unseat established bonds as our un-fixed, transitioning identities (Rogers 1951; Dexter 1996; Dryden and Thorne 1991; Johns 1996) buffet our surroundings, and we are 'weaned from previously unexamined patterns of behaviour' (Jourard 1971). I sometimes felt a kind of role confusion arising from moving through 'the crowded stage' (Johns 1996, p. 42) of people in my world, as I tried to find room for new parts of me and negotiate a subtly different way of relating in established friendships. There is a growing body of work on how insight training affects intimate partnerships (Guy 1987; Farber 1983; Cawkhill 2002; Collins 2008; Cowan 2012) but the complex bond of friendship is 'under-researched' (Adams and Blieszner 1994; Alhanati 2007) and only described anecdotally in Person-Centred literature, or as an adjunct to intimate partner studies. As my friendships are also hugely important bonds that provide sustenance which I need to practise (Guy 1987; Miller and Stiver 1997; Johns 1996; Comas-Diaz and Weiner 2013), it felt an important omission. I was conscious through training of multiple shifts taking place within my self-structure that I found difficult to articulate to friends outside the Counselling profession as I became a slightly quieter and more serious person in their midst. There was a combination of struggling to find a common language and also perhaps some fear that I might frighten them away. A rich closeness with others on my course, however, filled the gap and I became conscious of a movement away from some other friendships in a kind of 'creativity cycle of loosening and tightening' (Kelly 1955). It seemed that the gain in richness came at some cost.

Searching the literature began to shape the direction of the study as I engaged with resonant aspects that helped direct my interview schedule. Much of the literature describes hazards of practice that reflect the complexity of the work and the struggle to operate between the intensity of the therapeutic dyad and the outside world where trying to reach 'self-ideal congruence' (Guy 1987) seemed to require a balancing of a delicate emotional equation. I decided to research how other Person-Centred trainees managed this transition to a different way of relating and although I found some author accounts (e.g. Mearns 1997; Buchanan and Hughes 2000; Harding-Davies et al. 2004), I was struck by how few direct studies existed.

What the literature says
To place this piece of work into an allied research context and offer some background, I undertook a review of the core literature available to me in order to identify relevant themes and create a critical and analytical basis for further investigation. This familiarizing with existing work helped

me to note paucity and create my own area for exploration, but I stayed mindful of the need to maintain a healthy scepticism and a questioning stance and not to over-saturate myself, thus holding onto uniqueness and a space to generate ideas (McLeod 1993, p. 17). There is a balance to be maintained between being stimulated and informed, and being unbiased and open to surprise (West 2011). I found that there was a small body of work that looked at the impact of training to be a therapist on the extended private world of the therapist. However, there were no studies looking specifically at the lived-experience of change within friendships following Person-Centred training, apart from some anecdotal evidence within recent texts (e.g. Mearns 1997; Mearns and Thorne 2013; Buchanan and Hughes 2000, p. 91; Karter 2002), and a study by Dexter (1996) that touches on the social impact of Rogerian shaping. The existing work encompasses a small core of research studies (Cogan 1977; Guy 1987; Farber 1983; Skovholt and Ronnestad 1992; Truell 2001; Wright 2004; Alhanati 2007; Kennedy and Black 2010) which look at the intimate relationships of the therapist, but also examine the impact of training on the significant friendships of therapists. With the exception of Truell, these studies come from America and Canada, and are underpinned by heterogeneous psychotherapeutic traditions. I widened my search to include personal and professional development issues and transformative learning perspectives (Connor 1994; Mezirow 2000) which I felt would touch on some of the areas raised by my title and emerging themes from the literature. This included research looking at personal growth and the impact of personal development and change on the therapist (Skovholt and Ronnestad 1992; Dexter 1996; Mearns 1997; Harding-Davies et al. 2004). Despite it being an important area, there is relatively little specific, nuanced study, and even less within the last five years. Donati and Watts (2005), state that it continues to be a 'poorly defined area of training' and is one which is prey to 'conceptual fuzziness'. Connor (1994) suggests a rigorous course of training encourages 'profound' change, but it would seem that our detailed understanding of the tentacled impact 'outside the 50-minute hour' (Kennedy and Black 2010) on important social bonds, is relatively unexamined. Farber (1983, p. 174) notes this research gap has existed since Freud commented upon the 'dangers of analysis for the analyst'. In addition, I looked at studies examining impact of training on intimate partners (e.g. Fear 2004; Collins 2008; Cowan 2012). Other relevant literature reviewed, included the allied effects of working as a therapist, and how we develop our authentic selves within the therapeutic hour as we become neophyte practitioners. It felt important to get a feel for the literature examining the 'wounded Healer' (e.g. Jung 1951; Rippere and Williams 1985; Sussman 1992; Gladding 2004) and also that encompassing themes of impairment, burnout and isolation (e.g. Freudenberger and Robbins 1979; Kottler 2010; Barnett 2007); our motivations to train (Farber and Norcross 2005; Barnett 2007), and also at our existing psychological make-up (e.g. Henry, Sims and Spray 1973; Farber and Norcross 2005; Wheeler 2002; Mander 2004). I further explored the literature on friendship (e.g. Bukowski and Hoza 1989; Demir and Weitenkamp 2007; Helm 2010; Adams and Blieszner 1994) in order to understand its nature and bearing on our adult relational functioning. My aim was to get a feel for any of the potential concerns of my participants, and also to engage with the literature in a way that touched my own experiencing.

All therapy training demands a great deal from the participant but it can be argued that Person-Centred training asks the most of all. Owen (1993, p. 2) notes how 'the demands of the work on oneself and those at home, can be in conflict'. Mearns (1997, p. 113) talks of the emphasis on the personal and relational qualities of the Counsellor, and the 'daunting personal development objectives required'. He describes the 'greenhouse effect' of personal development creating a disparity and contrast in highly congruent relating between course members, and less congruent relating at home, and how 'it is impossible to go backwards' (p. 108). Change in Person-Centred therapy will be congruent with its core theoretical model. Dexter (1996, p. 89), in his critical review of the impact of Person-Centred Counsellor training, looks at the adoption of a fundamental philosophy shift inculcated through the learning of therapy which creates our perspective when viewing our fellow man. He suggests that trainees are not simply applying a set of skills that are picked up and then left at the counselling room door, but are asked at the most fundamental level, 'to develop trust as a replacement for responsibility'. Williams and Irving (1996, p. 165), in their study attempt to clarify thinking about differences between personal growth and development, stating that personal growth is a holistic concept, and 'Self actualization is a way of being, not simply a state of knowing'. They suggest that growth is not a learned theory but encompasses permanent change. Johns (1996, p. 59) echoes this, and suggests that trainees' change affects their 'whole person' and encompasses vast areas involving a 'unique pattern of moral, emotional, sexual, social and intellectual concerns'. Person-Centred training encompasses transformative learning perspectives (Cranton 1997; Mezirow 2000; Dirkx 2001) as we become emancipated from unconscious or unquestioning acceptance of what we have come to know about ourselves and our lives. We learn to make meaning, take ownership of our social roles, self-author, and take heed of our intuitive and unconscious processes. We can thus be seen to change fundamentally, and this ripples out into our private and social worlds. 'Also, psychotherapy ideologies have direct consequences as they can form the basis of a different way of life' (Owen 1993, p. 2).

Definitions of friendship include words such as trust, interpersonal bond, empathy, acceptance, honesty, altruism, understanding and compassion. Friendship is uniquely voluntary, dispositional and sociologically shaped. Friendship bonds can be considered to be relatively un-institutionalized, without standard rituals, norms or nomenclature to guide the partners or create a description. Friendship is thus difficult to study, or describe, as there is a lack of a cohesive theoretical basis (Adams and Blieszner 1994, p. 163; Nangle et al. 2003). Existing literature on friendship looks at the individual/personality and societal/structural factors that contribute to friendship bonding but there is a consensus that friendship patterns are likely to change as people make life course transitions (Allan and Adams 1989). Friendship bonds and therapeutic bonds thus have many words/features in common, but also some differences. Orlinsky (2012, p. 3) describes the therapeutic relationship in terms of a social bond. He embeds that relating within the sphere of personal life. Our social bonds (including 'best friends') are 'embedded in the individual's self, and from there radiate like the spokes of a wheel'. Thus he is saying that relating is at the heart of our work and friendships at the heart of our lives, and draws parallels to the quality of relating. 'There is of course, an important difference between the therapeutic relationship and other relationships in one's personal life. Ordinary personal relationships are mutual'. He goes on to say that there is a line between professional bonds and social bonds, and that the therapeutic relationship belongs to the therapist's 'professional life' and not his 'personal life'. Other definitions of friendship echo this mutuality and add choice and demographic compatibility as factors which differ from the characteristics of a therapeutic bond. Friendship is also linked to adjustment, quality of life/happiness and self-esteem (Demir and Weitenkamp 2007; Bukowski and Hoza 1989). However, there appears to be a gap in the literature describing this interface between our private and professional worlds, our therapeutic bonds and our friendship bonds – that space where they collide, and we must titrate our Person-Centred core conditioning to appropriately, and ethically, fit and fulfil our friendships and tune our relating thermostat. The Person-Centred ethos revolves around constructive personality change through relationship and Rogers (1961, p. 22) notes that '… it is a very paradoxical thing, that to the degree that each one of us is willing to change himself, then he finds not only himself changing, but he finds that other people to whom he relates are also changing'. Existing literature around the area of the private life of the therapist seemingly then, consists of descriptive accounts and personal experience of the phenomenon of relational/friendship change, but very little looks at just what happens when we are with our friends and working as Person-Centred practitioners.

Reviewing the literature illuminated two main 'cycles of interest': a series of studies from the 70s and 80s, and then those clustered around twenty years later. Earlier studies that specifically examine the impact of therapy training on friendship have relevance to the current post-modern era, but care needs to be taken when applying their findings to current Person-Centred training. Seashore (1995) noted his observations on the perils of professional development in a paper, where he stated that there may be 'a significant amount of conflict among those who liked you for what you were, not for what you are becoming'. Cogan's (1977) doctoral thesis looked at friendship amongst psychotherapists and noted how, at the time of training, friendships were felt as deep, intense and open. Participants reported that this was as a result of their work experience enabling a fuller investment in them. He noted, however, that after ten years of practice, they reported very few friendships, suggesting some kind of isolation and loss. Freudenberger and Robbins (1979), looking at the hazards of practice, suggested an increase in friendships with fellow therapists and a loss of friendship outside the profession, while other researchers in this era replicated themes of physical and psychic isolation (e.g. Deutch 1984; Goldberg 1986) and 'emotional tightness', as trainees learn to minimize their own responding (Malcolm 1980). Farber (1983, p. 175) used a large, heterogeneous sample of therapists to examine the extratherapeutic implications of practice on the therapist's world. It was heuristic in nature, and the results predicated on the notion that 'there exists a crucial connection between a person's work, and his behaviour and self-identity outside of the work environment'. His results indicate 'noticeable impact' across the spectrum of training schools, and a 'double-edged sword' theme echoes through the findings. The nature of insight training creates a 'psychological mindedness' which enriches friendship by fostering acceptance, depth, curiosity and sensitivity. However, the shadow side to this change suggests that this may also be pervasively consuming and 'interfere with natural, affective social interacting', including changes in disclosure levels (both ways), increased introspection, difficulty in setting aside a 'clinical persona', and a tendency to socialize less and with a smaller circle. Sixty-six per cent of the study cohort came from a psychoanalytic viewpoint, and findings thus cannot be easily applied to Person-Centred therapists. Farber (1983, p. 177) notes the limitations to a study trying to examine 'a huge, intangible area where it is difficult to get measures'. Guy (1987, p. 134) reiterates this theme of gain and loss within friendship as a result of being a therapist. His comprehensive literature review looks at all areas of the private world of the therapist, synthesizing available research. He suggests that 'personal assets and liabilities of being a psychotherapist, noticeably affect interactions with nearly everyone with whom the therapist experiences an intimate relationship'. The benefits of therapy training on friendship echo those found by Cogan (1977), and include an increased depth, intensity and openness to relating. The losses include emotional depletion caused by the intensive nature of the work leaving less time for the work of friendship, a corresponding inherent isolation, a blurring/ conflict of roles, loss of spontaneity and difficulty with mutuality. His conclusions pertain mainly to psychoanalytical training where he suggests that amongst therapists' friends, there may be a 'fear of being analyzed or manipulated' (p. 139). Some of Guy's (1987) observations are anecdotal and require further rigorous, empirical investigation. He suggests at one point that the 'hectic lifestyle' of the therapist may make him unavailable to friends, and that friends may expect 'free advice' leaving the therapist feeling 'used and exploited' (p. 138). He hints at role conflict and confusion, resulting from changed expectations/perceptions and shifted relational boundaries, but concludes that although these hazards of practice certainly impact on friendship, there is no 'conclusive data', and acknowledges that his findings are largely a result of 'conjecture and supposition' (p. 129).

The conclusions of recent studies looking at the impact of training on friendship seem to largely echo the earlier studies in finding a complex mix of gains and losses. However, rather than anecdotal descriptions of phenomena, they attempt to articulate the voice of the recent trainee. Skovholt and Ronnestad's (1992) model of Counsellor development places personal and professional development as the two strands that describe the broad learning process. Their fourteen themes note that 'across time, a professional's theoretical perspective and professional roles become increasingly consistent with his or her values, beliefs and personal life experience' (p. 1). It is a life-long process that may be erratic (p. 6). They further suggest that personal life, including peer relationships, influences professional functioning in both positive and adverse ways, but that the Counsellor's personal life relationships are a powerful influence (pp. 10–11). This offers a more integrated perspective in contrast to earlier work. Truell (2001, p. 3) used grounded theory and an in-depth semi-structured interviewing approach, to ask six recent Counselling graduates to comment on their training experiences. He reiterates earlier research into the losses around friendship experienced by seasoned therapists outlined by Guy (1987), but further suggests that newly qualified Counsellors are 'not only vulnerable to the same phenomena, but perhaps their problems are more intensified'. He suggests that they are less likely to have an integrated balance between their personal and professional lives. All six participants reported changes in their friendships. Five reported increased selectivity and distancing, one reported increased personal boundaries, and all noted a decrease in their number of friends. This was partly to do with not needing to 'please', outgrowing old patterns of relating, and the destabilizing effect associated with change. The positive aspects included the notion that the friendships that survived the training process were stronger, more intimate, and more meaningful than previously.

Buchanan and Hughes (2000, p. 91), in their compendium of Person-Centred trainee experiences, talk about the impact on friendship. They gained insights from a large number of trainees which include reported awareness of new patterns of relating at depth with peers on the course, that contrast with the quality of relating outside with friends. This 'eviction' from old ways of relating is a common theme throughout the literature, and its dual loss/gain outcome also seems to be a recurring theme in the description of both the gain in relational depth, and the loss of familiarity and consequent potential isolation with existing friendship. More recently, Wright (2004, p. 2) targeted 200 Counselling students from different training establishments, and asked them to describe their changes and consequent impact on relationships including friendship. Her findings are consistent with other contemporary studies (e.g. Buchanan and Hughes 2000; Karter 2002; Truell 2001; Alhanati 2007) in that the benefits were largely positive. However, she too noted the contrast between the congruent nature of course/peer relating, and how this 'could result in trainees becoming dissatisfied with their present friendships' outside.

Alhanati (2007) undertook a qualitative study of the personal lives of six therapists. Using thematic analysis, she asked them a series of questions about the impact of their work on various aspects of their lives including friendships. She noted a strong emergent theme of an 'intertwining of their personal and professional worlds' where her participants reported difficulty in separating out personal and professional lives into separate topics. She noted this as a unique finding which had been 'markedly omitted from the research literature to date'. However, her findings show a largely positive impact on friendship, with participants reporting stronger investment in meaningful friendships and a 'letting go' of more superficial ones. There was also an expressed desire for reciprocity and a shedding of friendships lacking mutuality. This suggests that old maladaptive friendship roles/patterns of behaviour were brought into awareness and were no longer as powerful, following insight training (Barnett 2007). Participants also reported better boundaries within interpersonal relationships and a greater acceptance, spirituality and compassion were also reported, as though life was viewed through a slightly different lens. Communication was better with enhanced tenderness, openness, warmth, listening and patience, culminating in enhanced 'presence'. A negative finding alluded to fatigue associated with the nature of therapeutic work, leaving participants depleted of energy to invest in friendship. However, Alhanati (2007) did not specify or ask her participants for their therapeutic orientation, and so it is difficult to assume that her findings are entirely reflective of Person-Centred trainee experience. However, embracing a post-modern constructionist approach to research, her participants' meaning–making holds truth in their worlds, and thus adds to a creative, open discussion.

Participants

Purposive sampling gave me access to participants with insight into my area of study, and despite extensive advertising at other training institutions, counselling organizations, the NHS and BACP online via poster and email, each of my subjects came via referral/snowballing. My criteria asked for practitioners with up to two years' experience to allow for recent reflection on their change process. However, I did not want to treat them as 'identikit'

(Smith et al. 2009, p. 50) and was prepared to be open to areas of divergence within the sample. I also felt a male perspective would be of value and one of my participants was able to offer this. The sample was aged between forty-five and sixty years, and two held a Master's degree in Counselling. All were currently working in both private and voluntary practice, and felt that the research area resonated sufficiently for them to connect with it.

Participant	Age Range	No. of Years qualified	Qualification	Place of Work
Sarah	40–50	1	Master's degree	Private Practice and School
Rachel	40–50	2	Diploma	FE College and Private Practice
Peter	50+	2	Master's degree	Private Practice
Anne	40–50	2	Diploma	Hospice

Table 3. Participants' details.

Sarah described the loss of two very close friends throughout and following training and the introspection of personal development is examined. Her narrative is framed very much around the core conditions as she explores the complexities of change on her friendships. Rachel examined the insight she has developed through her training and how this illuminates current friendship dynamics, particularly one long-standing complex friendship. Becoming more visible to others and increased expectations of in-depth relating, make up her story. Peter described feeling like two different people in relationship to friendship groups and examines how the core conditions work in existing friendships. He looks at how he marries together his worlds and the potential for enrichment. Anne talked about her core friendships and their importance in her world. Her role when being with a dying friend is reflected upon and also how her core friendships have moved with her changes.

Data collection

I devised an interview schedule of questions and then sent each participant a copy of the questions along with the consent form and information. The questions were:

- Do you feel your training has touched your friendships in any way?
- What have been the positives/gains?
- What have been the negatives/losses?
- Have you been aware of any ethical dilemmas within your friendships since training to be a Person-Centred therapist?
- How do you feel when your friends ask for support?
- How have you negotiated any changes around your friendships?
- Do your friends support your changes? Who is making the changes, and to what extent do they feel negotiated or forced?
- Do you think they understand the nature of your change?
- Have you noticed any changes in the make-up of your friendship group?
- Is there anything more you would like to add?

Findings

The data yielded a rich seam of themes and each seemed to bleed into the next, with sub-themes which straddled master themes. Table 4 below represents three master themes which I decided to focus on more fully. They seemed to be the most universal across my participants.

Overview of master themes with sub-themes
1. The Need for Enrichment and Depth in Friendship. 1.1 Relational depth and the need for intimacy. 1.2 Meaning of friendship. 1.3 Uniqueness of colleague-friend relating.
2. The Blending of the Professional and the Personal: A Collision of Worlds. 2.1 Role confusion/blending of selves. 2.2 Relational boundaries/on-off switch. 2.3 The continuum of the core conditions.
3. The Permanent and Personal Nature of Change and its Impact on Friendship. 3.1 Eviction from old ways of being. 3.2 No going back. 3.3 Outgrowth loss/gain.

Table 4. Emergent themes and sub-themes.

Master theme 1: The Need for Enrichment and Depth in Friendship

Sub-theme 1.1: Relational depth and the need for intimacy: All the participants were asked how their training had "'touched' their friendships, and later questions asked them to reflect on how they managed to negotiate the notion of support within friendship. Each person noticed how their expectations had shifted, and there was an expressed need for richer communication. This seemed to create both loss and

57

gain. Peter noticed how he sometimes felt a little outside his friendship group: *"It sometimes seems to me now that the conversation is around, particularly amongst the men but even amongst the women, is around relatively trivial things ... I kind of feel it's a bit superficial. There's also a loss of confidence ... there's some sort of response in me"* (Peter). Anne was able to reflect on which friends would be able to meet her at depth: *"It's funny how you realize 'horses for courses' ... who supports you, who is best in what. I know which friends are good for a great night out, and I know which friends I rely on if I was at death's door myself, you know?"* (Anne). She also expressed satisfaction in being asked to support her dying friend: *"She wanted to have the difficult conversations which now I've looked at it. I'm extremely privileged and proud that I could do that".* (Anne). The other three participants also echoed this feeling. All felt that being seen as someone able to offer trustworthy support felt *"an absolute positive"* (Sarah) and that they were *"touched"* (Peter). Sarah expressed the complexity of in-depth relating with friends: *"It's complex, but actually there's a simplicity as well, because there is only one way of being isn't there ... and you can't really change that"* (Sarah). She describes the gradual dissolving of a long-term friendship as her friend is unable to meet her need for congruence: *"I felt very uncomfortable being with somebody who isn't quite happy with the situation as it is, but isn't able to say anything"* (Sarah). But again, she demonstrates a light and shade within the change process wrought by training when talking about her friends who have stayed the course with her: *"There was a superficiality before. We didn't really go deep into feelings. Now, old friends that I've had for years and years, who have come on that journey with me, have changed ... we've changed"* (Sarah).

Sub-theme 1.2: Meaning of friendship: It felt almost artificial to delineate the sub-themes as they all delicately interweave. However, the language used when describing the meaning of friendship seemed noteworthy, and each participant spoke with language reflective of a deeper layer of felt-meaning, but also a need to find meaning in friendship following training: *"I get feelings of connectiveness which you could say, depending on your definition, are quite spiritual"* (Peter). *"When I did my course, it certainly made me reflect on the value of friendship. What this friendship meant to me and the incongruence part of it ... what I was harbouring that she didn't know about"* (Rachel). *"I wanted to do something more rewarding and completely different, but change everything else at the same time. So when you say: 'Did it touch your friendships?'... Yes it did in a massive way, because there was so much change. It made me appreciate the enormity of what I was doing and the importance of the friendships that I had"* (Anne). It seemed that training and the reflective nature of personal development, created a more global reflective illumination of friendship that both highlights difficulty and loss of friendship, and also throws into relief those more profound and resilient bonds.

Sub-theme 1.3: Uniqueness of colleague-friend relating: The notion that the participants were seeking more in-depth relating was borne out throughout each transcript, and elicited responses to questions about changes in the nature of their friendship group, which suggested that there was a shift towards friendships with counselling peers. *"So that friendship that I gained during training, has now probably replaced, and sort of added to some of the core people from before. That, I didn't appreciate, would happen"* (Anne). Peter, talking about a good friend who is also a Counsellor, hints at a kind of aloneness as a result of this shift: *"I'm quite often sitting in the pub thinking actually the only person I want to speak to is her, because I know as soon as we get going, it's going to be something more meaningful"* (Peter). A further feeling of sadness/loss is expressed by

Rachel: *"On the course, I've made a friend ... and when I compare the relationship I had with this person who I've become close to, to the friend I was mentioning before, it's such a different relationship and it makes me feel a bit sad really"* (Rachel). Again, light and shade is inherent. Sarah notes: *"On the course, I've made some wonderful friends ... everything you have shared has produced an honesty and even now we will get together and it is wonderful. The* (trust) *is quite precious to me because it hasn't happened a lot for me. It does with counselling friends ... but with actual friendships, it doesn't"* (Sarah). Both Sarah and Peter say that perceived depth is the binding feature: *"I've got some really good friends who are counsellors where I can share all that more intimate stuff, but actually in other spheres we haven't got so much in common"* (Peter). *"There's that sense of being in groups with people who are not even like-minded but who you share something really profound or fundamental or something really sensitive with"* (Sarah). There was both a sense of enrichment at the gain in meaningful friendships and also suggestion of the difficulties and threat to other friendships that may ensue.

Master theme 2: The Blending of the Professional and the Personal: The Collision of Worlds

Sub-theme 2.1: Role confusion/blending of selves: Although not directly framed as a question, but as a major component within my own research agenda, all four participants had noticed, on reflection, how friendships had become increasingly if subtly/intricately coloured by the inculcation of the core conditions from Person-Centred shaping. This is both positive: *"I think I have got a number of friendships where at some point or another, we've had some 'coun-sellory-like' discussions ... I make it very clear I'm not counselling them of course ... that has meant I have enjoyed some really nice deep discussions"* (Peter); and also confusing, as each

60

participant tried to work out 'who' they were being during friendship interactions: *"... there have been a couple of occasions when a friend has said something like, 'You sound just like a counsellor now'"* (Peter). Peter felt that he was *"easing in"*, but also that: *"at one point I was turning into two different people at the same time and I found it very, very difficult to switch between them"* (Peter). It seemed that 'role confusion' was not simply confined to the participants but also to their friends: *"There's this expectation that if you go out in a crowd ... that expectation from people that almost you have the answers ... which I clearly don't"* (Sarah). Each participant noticed a merging of roles in their interactions with their friends. In Anne's case, the circumstance of caring for her terminally ill close friend brought a *"crossing-over"* (Anne), that was very poignant: *"... conversations about everything else seemed to disappear and she would openly say she wanted to talk to me because she knew that I understood what it was like for people in her position because of the job I did ... but there was I, as her friend"* (Anne). This was very tough: *"But as a friend, I was having to be ... it was like there were two different people. I was very aware I was behaving like a counsellor in some of the conversations I had, because I was trying to keep myself together and not be the friend ..."* (Anne). The complex nature of change was very evident as each participant tried to wear their 'way of being' in the 'normal world': *"There were touches of moments when I thought we were quite close and I wanted this to be ... grown on, and occasionally it would be and I began to be aware that this was often when I was almost in counsellor mode, trying my hardest to sort of focus on those elements of unconditional respect ... She did respond to that"* (Rachel). Rachel goes on to say that she wasn't sure if *"that was really right"*, and Sarah too struggles with the interface between modes when describing her *"helping self"* within a friendship circle: *"I have to be conscious that I can't do that.*

Having said that, is it so different from being a friend? No. You are using the same conditions. So am I doing it? Probably. When I think about it, yes I am" (Sarah).

Sub-theme: Relational boundaries/on-off switch: My question about ethical boundaries elicited some responses which further echoed the complexity of being trained and the differences between friendship-relating and therapeutic-relating. Sarah describes how she tries to process and manage this: *"I try to* (create boundaries), *but of course it's very difficult because all my good friends know what I do. So that can't be boundaried ... it's there"* (Sarah). *"There is definitely a mutuality, but there is also a sense of ... professionalism ... I do try not to be anything people expect me to be. I just want to have a drink and be with my friends. I don't know about easy, but it's doable"* (Sarah). Peter explores the subtle differences between friends and clients as a way of delineating his boundaries: *"With a friend, I do have an agenda unlike if I was a counsellor, so I'm interested in them and so it means I can be much more analytical. I can ask questions ... I suppose play with psychology which you know interests me which you can't do when you are counselling and I would throw myself more into it ... perhaps I might spin off and talk about similar experiences"* (Peter). Peter seemed clearer about his boundaries than perhaps the other participants: *"I can't see how there could possibly be an ethical line in using the core conditions outside of counselling"* (Peter). Anne also felt some clarity in certain situations about how to create boundaries: *"If it did cross-over, I wouldn't have an issue saying it"* (Anne). However, she felt more difficulty when working through the delicate ethics of caring for her dying friend: *"Here it was, mirroring the issues with confidentiality ... everything about boundaries was all over the place because she was my friend ..."* (Anne). Rachel also felt less secure with boundaries and managing her 'on-off switch': *"There was a certain way of being* *there, which I'd stepped out of something and into something else. I felt that shift, it felt in a way that I'd stepped out of the friendship and was in a different role"* (Rachel). All the participants seemed to be aware of some conflicts and difficulties and the process of managing them was ongoing and reflective of the exploration/integration stage that each was working through.

Sub-theme 2.3: The continuum of the core conditions: A sub-theme that blends through all the others within this super-ordinate bracket, was how the cornerstone of Person-Centredness, the core conditions, were impacting on friendship. Sarah, in particular, very much framed her narrative using the core conditions as a benchmark for relating. Congruence, for her, was an embedded shift/ influence: *"The other thing was, I guess, the congruence and the fact that I could only be a certain way now"* (Sarah). *"Now it's there, and if I don't say it, it sits with me. I don't know where to put it so it has to come out"* (Sarah). Again, Peter was more circumspect when asked about any losses in friendship since training: *"I can't really think of any sort of mechanism whereby that might happen, because if one is sustaining a relationship more, with an awareness of the core conditions and using them perhaps, I can't see how that would prise anything out of the relationship"* (Peter). Nevertheless, Peter too noticed on further reflection, how perhaps he felt sometimes more vulnerable: *"I have found that in making myself more sensitive to others, I have become more sensitive to things happening to me"* (Peter). It seemed that the core conditions when part of friendship dynamics also created some positive ripple effects in friends: *"When friends ask for help, it just feels ... natural, normal ... they just feel they can have an open and honest conversation"* (Anne). However, it also seemed to create some risk, and Rachel reflected on how one of her close friends may have struggled: *"I think you could* say that being congruent didn't suit everyone" (Rachel). It seemed that those more fragile/ambivalent friendships formed before training, were the ones that were most threatened during, and following, training. However, the dominant feeling from the participants was one of enrichment in friendship, and positive benefit across the more secure friendships: "I think some of what I've been through, confrontation isn't a bad thing. So it's all about honesty" (Anne). "I am definitely a lot more relaxed with my friends … but the honesty is still possibly the same and you know, the core conditions are still there … still the same" (Sarah). Sarah noticed how this enabled her friends to feel safe enough to ask for support: "There's a sense of responsibility there for sure, but overriding, that there's a real sense of I'm pleased that they can ask me … whether that comes from the helping side of me … it's about listening. How easy is that but how often does it happen?" (Sarah).

Master theme 3: The Permanent and Personal Nature of Change and its Impact on Friendship

All four participants struggled to communicate their changes to their friends who had possibly noticed but were not "in on it" (Rachel). Indeed each felt the complexity of personal development almost as hard to understand for themselves: "I don't understand it properly myself" (Sarah).

Sub-theme 3.1: Eviction from old ways of being: An illumination of old patterns of relating was one of the powerful sequelae of training: "It made me realize I was doing certain things for the wrong reasons, and that I didn't have to do them at all" (Rachel). Rachel described how "challenging" this was to others' notions of her previous "agreeable" relating style, but that it made her "accept" herself and "enjoy other people" in new ways. However, again the loss/gain nature of change was apparent, and for Peter, his world view was profoundly altered by training: *"It kind of was a bit of a shock to be honest ... not a shock that suddenly hit me, but over a period of months you know, that really built up to be a major challenge to my ... how I felt about the world really"* (Peter). He described feeling kind of a social *"loss of confidence"* when in company with friends who were not on his *"wavelength"*, and also, like Sarah, struggled with trying to communicate this: *"I haven't been able to try and describe them to them. It kind of seems a bit personal, a bit spiritual ..."* (Peter). *"It's made me feel a bit sad about not actually being able to share something that's very important and precious to me with some of my closest friends"* (Peter). Anne notes how her needs have changed: *"But to me, friendships, and what I want from a friendship, is now very different where I am in my life now"* (Anne). Sarah, too, notes how she has different needs and that this has expedited the end of friendship: *"That friendship has gone I would say, because of the counselling, or because of the way I have changed"* (Sarah). All four participants were aware of the permanent shifts that had taken place, and the paradoxical push-pull of complexity/simplicity where life seemed *"so much easier before"* (Sarah). And yet, there was an integrity and honesty to friendship that was perhaps missing previously.

Sub-theme 3.2: No going back: *"You can't un-learn something"* (Sarah). There was a real sense that despite the losses inherent in change, the gains to friendship in being in the world as a Counsellor were permanent and worthwhile: *"Whilst I risk my friendships ... parts of them ... it has to be, because I couldn't go back to where I was. There is no way of going back there"* (Sarah). Rachel talks about her tendency to rescue that has been a feature of pre-training relating: *"I cannot do that. I used to when I was younger ... my friends needed something, I was there in a flash. I can't do that now"* (Rachel). Anne communicated her sense of empowerment: *"I'm now fully* *aware that it's all my choice, and I'm doing what I want to do"* (Anne); and Peter, a deeply felt congruence: *"I think how I was turning into a counsellor felt more consistent with my true being"*, even if in so doing, he felt it necessary to *"jettison"* a group of friends.

Sub-theme: Outgrowth loss/gain: Linked into the other sub-themes, each participant expressed feelings of a world left behind – although as with the other themes, there were areas of divergence amongst them. Out of the four, Anne's core friendship group remained the most stable, and she very much felt that *"they've been through it **with** me"*. Rachel describes how she feels a difference in emotional investment: *"I suppose what I'm noticing is that the more I'm trying to give and trying maybe to facilitate, I don't feel that I'm getting that back"* (Rachel). *"Friendships went, because they couldn't relate to me in the same way and I probably haven't got time to relate to them ..."* (Rachel). Peter echoes this kind of gulf: *"It's really hard to describe the sort of impact a counselling course has on someone who doesn't really, hasn't really, thought of that sort of thing"* (Peter). Sarah expressed a feeling that overall, her level of trust *"has gone down"* in her friends, and differentiated between her counselling friendships in the sense that she could now identify who she felt safe with. Anne sums up the reorganization of friendship dynamics and touches on the subtle shifts and nuanced changes involved in insight training evolution: *"If something massive happened in my life then I know who would still want to be part of my life and who I could count on ... so things have evolved and changed. They get dragged into different positions. So, I'm still in the mix with people, I still call them my close friends but they all play a different part in it"* (Anne). Throughout their gradual transformation, all four participants felt parallel shifts amongst friendship groups that were multilayered and subtle. The overall sense was of positive enrichment within friendship bonds which nevertheless involved loss of friends who were unable to stay with the process. There was also a sense of the irreversibility of this and a coming to terms with endings. Identity and 'way of being' also seemed to be something to be negotiated. A blending/confusion was noted which may be reflective of the relatively recent time since training. The findings were consistent with other similar research in that all four partici-pants experienced a destabilization in their private friendship world following training, which resulted in a complex mix of losses and gains. There was a powerful sense of movement in all friendship bonds that echoed the participants' personal development and a sense of the complexity of the task of integrating the worlds.

Discussion

There is no doubt that training to be a Person-Centred therapist has altered the timbre of the friendships of the participants in this study, and this chimes with Mearns (1997, p. 108), who notes that congruence, and the 'substantial incongruence' of the 'real world', can create a kind of relational no-man's-land for the trainee, whereby they can move neither to the other side, nor indeed go backwards. Person-Centred training is a complex process (Johns 1996; Mearns and Thorne 2013), interwoven with natural maturation (Brown 1981) that creates a very delicate and subtle re-organization/transformation (Mezirow 2000) of identity that has somehow got to be *"eased in"* (Peter) to everyday life. One outcome of a Rogerian training has been described as inducing a kind of 'dynamic disequilibrium' (Hall et al. 1999, p. 9). Friendship too, is a 'dance of intimacy' where 'being who we are, requires that we can talk openly about things that are important to us' (Lerner 1989, p. 3). As a concept to define, friendship is complicated and also affected by natural life-course changes outside of training (Adams and Blieszner 1994). Whilst setting myself a difficult task to try and understand the nature of that dance, I allowed the participants to freely choose those friendship bonds they wished to examine, and thus self-define, what were, to them, very personal bonds. My findings echo much of the existing work in that for each of the participants, all of whom are at 'novice professional phase' (Ronnestad and Skovholt 2003), there have been both losses and gains in their private lives and friendship dynamics (Cogan 1977; Farber 1983; Guy 1987).

Adams and Blieszner (1994) delineate a framework on which to examine friendship which comprises three interacting elements that operate at both dyadic and network levels of friendship. They include 'structure' (the form of the ties linking an individual's friends, solidarity and similarity), 'phases' (the formation, maintenance and dissolution of friendship dyads and of clusters of friends within networks) and 'interactive processes' (thoughts, feelings and behaviours involved in acting as friends). From the transcripts, it is evident that Person-Centred training impacts each element, with perhaps the 'phases' element being the most notable. It seems that training has the potential to destabilize and create *"big shifts"* (Rachel) within the maintenance phase of an established dyad, whereby decisions are made 'whether to retain the friendship at its current level of solidarity, change it to a higher or lower level of involvement, engage in different activities all together, dissolve the friendship, display indifference to it' (Hays 1989). Connor (1994, p. 29) suggests that in order to fulfil the requirements of training, one must inculcate the ethos of the core theoretical model offered, and that a 'good course' leads to 'profound change'.

Dexter (1996, p. 80) calls this adoption of a 'new philosophy', a 'powerful phenomenon', and suggests that 'it is difficult to imagine other subjects having so much potential impact on the student's life'. The heartfelt adoption of the Person-Centred ethos focusing on the core conditions by all four participants, certainly bears this out.

One of the most powerful feelings from the transcripts (which became a master theme) was the increased need for enrichment and depth as a central feature of friendship. This quest for more intense and intimate encounters, paradoxically both enhanced friendship and also expedited the dissolution of friendship. It seemed that being exposed during training and following it, to relationships that operate beyond presentational level that are 'utterly committed to congruence', and where the thriving trainees' 'endeavour is so firmly tied to who the therapist is a person' (Mearns and Cooper 2005, p. 137), creates a feeling/need for all communication to carry meaning; 'Indeed we may, for a time, become voracious feeders on encounter having been starved for so long' (Mearns and Cooper 2005, p. 147). Each participant expressed this in their own way, from Peter's *"itching to get on to some deeper stuff"*, to Rachel's soul searching; *"What does this relationship mean? What's it all about?"*. McAucliffe's (2002) study, asking Counselling students what personal changes they most noticed as a consequence of training, described an increased valuing of dialogue, reflexivity and autonomy, and it certainly felt that the participants also needed this from friendship. The sub-themes in this master theme-set, as well as illustrating the need for depth and meaning, also include the observation that friendships with fellow Counsellors often met these needs more fully. All four participants noticed that their friendship groups had shifted, and either a peer trainee or another Counsellor had assumed an important space within their friendship world. This fits in with both other anecdotal evidence (e.g. Buchanan and Hughes 2000, p. 91), and research. Truell (2001) noted that trainees became more selective about which friends they wanted to spend time with, but unlike the participants in this study, framed this as a stressor. Guy and Liaboe (1986) noted that Counsellors experienced difficulties with their ability to relate meaningfully with friends. However, all four participants communicated that the addition of these friends who could meet them at depth, added to what Kennedy and Black (2010, p. 428) describe as a 'richer life', and hint at Maslow's (1943) 'Good life'. Nevertheless, the gain/loss nature of the extant literature is reflected within the transcripts too: *"Other friends went, because they couldn't relate to me in the same way"* (Rachel). All four participants expressed sadness as the 'angle-poise' of training shone on their more superficial alliances, and ties were loosened. All four substantiated the findings from other studies of smaller friendship groups and increased friendship selectivity (e.g. Cogan 1977; Truell 2001; Alhanati 2007; Buchanan and Hughes 2000). I think, for me, one of the most resonant themes to emerge from this study, was the notion of the blending of the personal and professional selves, and the resultant collisions and role confusion as the *"the two merge"* (Sarah). Alhanati (2007), too, cited this as an unexpected main theme in her study. As Stevens (1996, p. 2) notes, the self is a profoundly social phenomenon, and each of us 'inhabits a distinctive social world of lived-experience. We are conscious of being, and are seen by others as being a *particular person'*. Each of our friendships has a unique hue, and when we change, so does the shading of that hue as we add a further dimension of self to the mix. Furthermore, 'friendship and counselling enjoy a complex and paradoxical relationship' (Russell and Dexter 2008, p. 530). Each participant disclosed instances of role confusion when in helping situations with friends. Rogers (1980) describes the Person-Centred ethos as 'quietly subversive' and almost a revolutionary 'social mediator'. As a microcosm of society, our friendship networks seemingly undergo 'quiet' mediation as we train. When asked whether clients could become friends, Mearns and Thorne (2013, p. 210) point out that with the Person-Centred approach, the centrality of power sharing and mutuality mean that it is more like a friendship than any other form of therapy, and feel that with negotiated responsibility, it is possible. However, it is this 'grey area' negotiation of a dual relationship with friends that the participants discovered as difficult. When the received wisdom of this orientation is that we use our 'person' and not our 'role' (Mearns and Thorne 2013, p. 215), it is seemingly harder to navigate boundaries not clearly delineated by a job description.

All the participants, however, explored ways of integrating their counselling selves, and managing the fine line between helping, and counselling, friends. Lynch (2002, p. 74) in his work on pastoral counselling, describes how closely related counselling and friendship can be, and talks of pastoral counselling as a kind of 'moderated friendship'. Aristotle (1990) postulated that the highest form of friendship is 'a friendship of virtue'. His description shares many counselling characteristics, including 'fundamental love and regard for each other'. It seemed that each participant found a way of counselling friends that allowed for safe, contracted exchanges that preserved the essence of friendship, integrity and boundaries. Anne, in particular, when supporting her dying friend, held boundaries, preserved confidentiality, but remained herself. Russell and Dexter (2008, p. 54) when looking at the 'un-shod' Counsellor, i.e. in an out of office scenario, argue that through 'trust and negotiation', this is entirely possible. 'Indeed, our prior knowledge of each other challenges us to demonstrate a very clear negotiated understanding without contamination'. They liken the notion of counselling friends to peer triad work in training. This was not straightforward for any of the participants, however, and the delicacy and self-awareness required when trying to contract outside the therapy room, led to some identity confusion and perhaps 'contamination': *"You know, we don't sit and contract, but actually you kind of do"* (Sarah). Sarah struggled with confidentiality, and with the notion that disclosure from a friend could not be shared even with her husband. This is something all the participants were working through, and echoes some of the literature on the isolation of confidentiality (Egan 1973; Tamura et al. 1996). Linked into this, the management of relational boundaries became a further sub-theme encompassing the way the participants managed their 'on-off switches' (Farber 1983). *"I try to* (create boundaries), *but of course it's very difficult, because all my good friends know what I do. So that can't be boundaried. It's there"* (Sarah). However, unlike the groundswell of earlier literature findings that 'psychological mindedness' (Farber 1983, p. 178) became a way of life, making it difficult to switch off, and that 'the job possesses the man' (Terkel 1972), the four participants managed the titration most of the time; *"it's definitely do-able"* (Sarah). Peter delineated social gatherings where *"quite often a glass of wine would be involved"*, but all were aware that some of their friends were less able to manage boundaries, and all expressed instances where they were looked to, to provide answers. A feeling I got from the participants, was that their ability to manage, and be aware of, boundary issues, although complex and ongoing, helped them create more deep and meaningful bonds (Guy et al. 1987), and avoid hazards such as depletion and isolation (Freudenberger and Robbins 1979). However, as each interview progressed it seemed to unfurl further dilemmas that were previously on their edge of awareness, and each participant reflected on the multilayered tasks of change. This may be a reflection of their relatively recent entry into a Counselling role, and reiterates Truell's (2001) similar finding, that newly qualified Counsellors had not perhaps integrated the personal/professional balance as well as more seasoned therapists. It is also possibly a reflection of the lifelong complicated, multifaceted process of interaction and transition, where 'boundaries, like so much else in the Person-Centred tradition, are not simply imposed, but explored and agreed' (Mearns and Thorne 2013).

A further sub-theme within this 'collision of worlds', was the continuum of use of the core conditions through everyday life and how they had come to define thinking and relating for the participants. Each participant noticed an impact on both themselves and on their friends as they became an embedded part of their everyday being and communicating. It seemed that the participants' friends could 'catch the empathic ability' (Mearns and Thorne 2013, p. 215) in a way that clients could from a strong therapeutic bond. Increased acceptance and tolerance of friends was expressed as a positive outcome of training, as empathy and unconditional regard became more conscious processes. It would seem inevitable that enhanced psychological contact and openness with friends was a natural consequence of this, as trainees' parallel growth occurred as a consequence of these 'necessary and sufficient conditions' (Rogers 1961). This echoed similar findings from other studies (e.g. Williams and Irving 1996; Dexter 1996; Truell 2001; Alhanati 2007). However, an unexpected finding was that when their friends asked for support, which seemed to happen more readily, each participant felt something like satisfaction. Responses ranged from *"touched"* (Peter), *"privileged"* (Anne) *"pleased ... natural"* (Sarah) and *"fine"* (Rachel), although of the four, Rachel was most conscious of guarding against being 'used'. Anne's touching account of being entrusted to manage her friend's dying, as both a friend and a Counsellor, despite being extremely harrowing to negotiate, was described by Anne as the *"ultimate"* form of friendship. Each accepted that their new roles would alter the rules in the sense that they were now recognized as 'skilled' helpers, even if they had always seen themselves inclined that way before training, as each participant did (Guy 1987; Farber et al. 2005; Barnett 2007). This perhaps reflected an enhanced confidence, an ability to manage the boundaries, and also that there is something about being a Person-Centred Counsellor that is inevitably carried through to everyday life, and possibly more so than other forms of counselling. This resonates with Cramer's work which correlates enhanced self-esteem, with perceived core conditions within friendship (Cramer 1994). As with the other themes, this one also created casualties where *"I think you could say, congruence didn't suit everyone"* (Rachel). The need for greater congruence, out of all the core conditions, seemed for all the participants to be the most uncompromising change for them within friendships and cited most often as the most challenging to negotiate. This reflects its status as 'one of the most complex issues to study within the Person-Centred Approach' (Granfanaki 2001), and the most difficult to inhabit (Greenberg and Geller 2001; Omylinska-Thurston and James 2011). This facet certainly seemed to offer the most high-risk challenge to established friendships.

The third master theme arising from the participants' narratives, was how training was a permanent, but very personal, process, and the fallout from being 'evicted' from old ways of relating had an impact on friendships, in the sense that it was very difficult to communicate to someone outside, the very intricate internal shifts that had taken place. This meant that friendships were destabilized through unannounced/unspoken power shifts and outgrowth that even the participants struggled to understand (Wright 2004; Johns 1996; Skovholt and Ronnestad 1992; Mearns 1997; Guy 1987). Rachel, in particular, noticed threat as a consequence of her growing self-awareness and need to be more visible to a close friend. This has led to her re-assessing this long-standing friendship that is certainly in jeopardy. Each participant felt the risks and sadness as a result of being unable to articulate their movement that felt so *"personal"* and *"spiritual"* (Peter). Both Peter and Sarah expressed more seismic changes, that fit in with the literature on trans-formative change (e.g. Mezirow 2000; Connor 1994; Alhanati 2007), where they became 'critically aware of (their) own tacit assumptions and expectations, and those of others' (Mezirow 2000, p. 4). Sarah's loss of two major relationships, and Peter's *"shock"* at the strength of his new *"world view"* really destabilized their friendship networks, culminating in Peter's case in a *"jettisoning"* of both a previous career and the associated friendships. Again, as in nearly all the other studies (e.g. Guy 1987; Alhanati 2007; Truell 2001; Wright 2004), as well as the losses, there were also gains to becoming 'different' in relationship. An enjoyment and appreciation of what friendships beyond counselling offered, ran through all the transcripts as the participants gained insight into both themselves and others. Anne's training has made her a *"different person"*, but she nevertheless, perhaps more than the other three, was able to carry her core friends through training. The permanence of change came through a sense of there being 'no going back'. With each participant, I felt that they couldn't reverse the processes of change and were accepting of the losses that may occur as a result: *"I could only be a certain way now and it was **this** way"* (Sarah). There was a real sense of 'this is me now' and a commitment to 'authentic living' (Mearns and Thorne 2013, p. 62).

The final sub-theme, which perhaps encompasses all the others, is the notion of 'outgrowth'. Much of the early literature on the impact of training on friendship focuses on such 'ubiquitous stressors' (Brady et al. 1995) as depletion, isolation, burnout and 'psychological mindedness', creating a distance between therapist and friend (Freudenberger and Robbins 1979; Farber 1983); and the enclosed, private nature of therapy, making sharing its challenges with non-therapist friends, complex (Speigel 1990; Thorenson et al. 1989). It would seem that the participants in this study have not really expressed the former as being major difficulties, although there was sometimes a sub-textual sense that they were 'there'. They were certainly not prompted by the questions asked. The egalitarian nature of Person-Centredness, with its embeddedness in the person as a 'way of being', possibly precludes a skill-distancing and guards against professional hazards in that sense. More recent studies have perhaps been more resonant of this study and its findings, whereby personal development and the ability to communicate at depth have perhaps left some friendships behind (Mearns 1997; Truell 2001; Wright 2004). A kind of accelerated maturation was described, that whilst creating greater tolerance, acceptance and enrichment, has also culminated in the loss, or demotion, of long-standing friendships for Sarah and Rachel, and the movement away from groups of friends for Peter. *"They've seen the change, but I don't think they're in on it"* (Rachel). The master themes represent the most convergent experiences of the four participants. As 'unique selves' (Mearns and Thorne 2013, p. 58) there were some findings that were special to each one, that perhaps deserve discussion. For Rachel there was need to be *"seen"* and *"heard"* that came from her greater self-awareness, and which made her want to re-evaluate one particularly difficult friendship and work at it. This echoed findings by Buchanan and Hughes (2000, p. 91) that trainees are able to 'recreate and reinforce the old friendships with a greater degree of openness to them', although this friendship was nevertheless struggling to survive as her friend struggled to match this openness. Sarah lost perhaps most with her established friendships, and unlike Rachel, felt that *"generally trust has gone down"*. Anne, uniquely, had kept her core friendship group fully intact, although *"things have evolved and changed ... they get dragged into different positions"*. She felt that because she was single and had no children, her friendships were centrally important: *"They've been through it with me, you see?"*. Peter, described a powerful kind of response when out with his non-counselling friends, that suggested that he was somehow out of step and incongruent, an ensuing loss of *"social confidence"* that, to him, felt quite negative. His seemed a particularly strong need to be congruent and 'in contact' with his friends, but possibly came closer than the female participants to 'psychic isolation' where 'constant immersion in a world replete with psychopathology and dysfunction isolates' (Brady et al. 1995), and may create some separateness (Thorenson et al. 1989).

Conclusion

Whilst not aiming to generalize my findings, the data collected is nevertheless dependent on the material offered by my participants and also on my skill in both collection and analysis. Different researchers may create different interpretations (Denzin and Lincoln 2005). The unique, complex nature of change, and limitations of language and conceptual heterogeneity in describing transitions, also adds a layer of difficulty to conducting the study. Although this has the added layer of richness from interpretation and critical thinking, it also adds an inherent tension to this type of study. This has been a small-scale, qualitative study that has attempted, by engaging the hermeneutics of empathy and questioning (Smith et al. 2009), to begin to unravel the lived-experience of Person-Centred trainees' change on their friendships, and to try and move away from assumption and towards the 'essence' (Husserl 1927) of what it feels like to manage the potential conflicts and paradoxes within this transition, when the outside world 'seems' to remain the same. My findings echo existing themes in other research, in that the participants experienced, within their friendships, a complex array of losses. These encompassed notions of outgrowth, and eviction from old patterns of relating in friendship, that felt destabilizing. However, the powerful gains, including enrichment, authenticity and satisfaction from offering 'ultimate' parts of self, were felt as permanent movements towards more meaningful relating and deeper bonds (Guy 1987; Truell 2001; Alhanati 2007); and this 'quiet revolution' (Rogers 1980) seemingly spread out to those friends who could 'stay the course'. This study has particularly noted the affect from the alchemy of the core conditions, most especially 'congruence'. Uncompromising, 'open and intimate' relating (Buchanan and Hughes 2000, p. 91), has been one of the most unifying outcomes and suggests, for these participants, that Person-Centred training really has become a part of 'being' outside the therapy room. Nevertheless, the collision of worlds, and subtle role confusion as the personal and professional are integrated, can feel lonely and difficult, and the 'retrospective understanding of superficiality' (Buchanan and Hughes 2000) created friendship casualties. The stage of training/time since qualification may all be factors in colouring our friendship landscape, and the complexity of deconstructing the friendship bond (Nangle et al. 2003) and interpreting another's life-world, make drawing conclusions tentative. These have been 'my' meanings and contribution (Etherington 2004).

Person-Centred therapy effectiveness is dependent on the effectiveness of the therapist (Mearns and Thorne 2013), and therapy research should make some contribution to better therapeutic practice' (West 2011). The 'friendship research' overwhelmingly agrees that friendship is 'life enhancing' (Helm 2010). We need our friends (both peer and non-Counsellor), and they are centrally important in nourishing us (Guggenbuhl-Craig 1979; Guy and Liaboe 1986; Johns 1996; Demir and Weitenkamp 2007; Comas-Diaz and Weiner 2013). Further, our struggles to integrate transition into our personal world mirror those of our clients. Detailed, rigorous understanding of our own process, and the development of strategies to manage these transitions in the context of our friendships, can only benefit our clients; including strategies in training courses, as informed elements of personal development and the structured dissemination of findings, would contribute to both Counsellor and client well-being.

CHAPTER THREE

THE EXPERIENCES OF PET OWNERS' WELL-BEING GAINED THROUGH THEIR RELATIONSHIPS WITH THEIR COMPANION ANIMALS

Jennifer Jane Johnson

Introduction

Within this small-scale research project, my aim is to investigate the well-being significance of the experiences of relating to a companion animal. I am particularly interested in the ways in which the human–animal relationship enhances well-being. In my personal life, I have noticed that after the daily miserable commute to work, I could simply imagine my dog and my gloom lifted. Unexpectedly I would actually smile, lending physical proof that my dog was improving my mood from forty miles away. I tried substituting thoughts of human loved-ones, but nothing else worked consistently well in effecting the positive change. Thoughts of human loved-ones soon inspired complex concerns, whereas thinking about my dog was uncomplicated and instantly cheering. The feelings of peace and calm impressed me. Low mood, stress, anxiety and depression affect many of the callers to Samaritans where I volunteer, as well as the clients I work with in a medical centre as a Person-Centred Counsellor. Factors in people's lives that might provide a buffer, or relief to distress, are worthwhile investigating. Hence the research question which I am addressing in this study is: How does the relationship with companion animals contribute to people's well-being?

By 'well-being' I mean happiness, contentment and mental good health. Although I prefer the term 'companion animal' to the term 'pet', which 'is often associated with the animal being seen as simply an object or a possession' (Society for Companion Animal Studies 2013a), for reasons of clarity and variety I will use both terms in this study.

It is the 'everyday experience' that particularly interests me, the taken-for-granted aspects of the relationship that people have with their companion animals. Through my study, I am seeking to bring into awareness the emotional gifts that people receive through their connection with an animal. It is the unique essence of these relationships that I wish to capture.

Our relationship with domestic animals dates back to early hunting communities 500,000 years ago. In later human history there is evidence of companion animal ownership in ancient Egyptian, Greek, Roman and Chinese civilizations (Bradshaw 2011, 2013; Robinson 1995; Serpell 1995). The human–animal relationship is embedded in our cultural, social and historical context. From childhood, our stories are filled with animal figures in a multitude of forms. The world's cultures, both past and present, feature animals as status symbols and helpers as well as companions (Franklin 1999; Podberscek et al. 2000). Our capacity to interact effectively with dogs and horses in particular, allows us to employ them in an impressive number of areas, such as rescue, military, policing, sport, entertainment, scientific research, child development, medical therapies and support for people with disabilities (Robinson 1995). These working roles often coexist with the companion role. However, companionship is the most common reason for pet ownership in western societies with almost a third of UK households owning a dog or a cat (FEDIAF 2012). The companion bond has been shown to provide significant benefits both medically and socially (Society for Companion Animal Studies 2013b). Pet ownership in British contemporary society has become widely accepted as beneficial:

> While in the 1960s close relationship with a pet was widely considered dissocial and the cause for some concern, in the 1990s the development of very close, human-styled relationships with animals is normative and, indeed, therapeutic (Franklin 1999, p. 5).

With such rapid changes in attitude within our society (Bradshaw 2011, 2013; Fogle 1983; Serpell 1995), Counsellors might fail to consider the significance of the human–animal bond for their clients (Noonan 2008; Owen 2008; Sable 2013; Walsh 2009a; Wells 2011; Vining 2003). It is clear that some people's well-being can be enhanced through their relationship with a companion animal (Society for Companion Animal Studies 2013b). Yet I anticipate that looking in-depth at individual experiences will provide a source of rich material. Because my small-scale study focuses on the ordinary, everyday experience of people, I have chosen a phenomenological approach (Silverman 2010) using qualitative methods (Maykut and Morehouse 1994).

I am aware that I come to the topic with particular biases, and I will persevere to bracket these off during the process (Willig 2008; Denscombe 2014). Firstly, my own experience leads me to believe that there is a unique joy to be found in the relationship between human and animal, and that it can confer well-being. Secondly, as a dog owner, I want to give unbiased attention to other companion animals within my study. Thirdly, I believe that some people are inclined to underestimate the importance of the relationship, at least when expressing themselves to others. As Counsellors, we work with clients to explore how they experience the world, naturally focusing on human relationships both past and present. I want to explore my suspicion that, within the counselling relationship, clients might minimize, or even ignore, animal relationships that can be powerful and rich. This minimizing might happen through a natural inclination to filter out these bonds because they involve non-humans and therefore may seem trivial, or perhaps because people feel inhibited about discussing their importance.

What the literature says

> Not so long ago, the idea of studying social relationships between humans and other animals would have been regarded as tantamount to heresy. In Europe, until the early modern period, animals were viewed as irrational beings placed on earth solely for the economic benefit of mankind, and most scholars would have insisted that affectionate relationships between people and animals were not only distasteful but depraved. Happily those days are now gone (Podberscek et al. 2000).

It was the mid-twentieth century when 'those days' began to recede, because the benefits for people from their relationships with companion animals captured the interest of academics. Leading the way were Veterinary Scientists, joined by scholars from Medicine, Psychology, Sociology, Anthropology, Zoology, Philosophy, Economics, Ecology, Education, Art and Literature. Indeed there is now a growing area of study, Anthrozoology, which combines a number of these disciplines in order to focus on the study of the Human–animal Interactions (HAI) and the human–animal bond (HAB). The idea that we benefit from keeping pets is not entirely new in British culture (Franklin 1999). William Turk, an eighteenth-century Quaker philanthropist, observed that the severe mental disorders of patients were relieved when the courtyards of the York Retreat asylum that he ran were stocked with small domestic animals, as well as seagulls and hawks (Franklin 1999; Robinson 1995; Wells 2011). In English asylums, this therapeutic use of animals continued throughout the nineteenth century in order to provide a 'less hostile, and more attractive, environment' (Wells 2011, p. 172). Animals were also valued for their effects on physical health. Indeed, in the late nineteenth century, Florence Nightingale was struck by the pleasure that long-term patients gained from the presence of a bird (Wells 2011). The most notable pioneer of ethology was Konrad Lorenz (2002), whose book *Man Meets Dog* was first published in German in 1949, and translated into English in 1954. The English translation is still selling well, even though many of these scientific theories have been superseded. It is valued for what Lorenz tells of the human–animal bond that he explores through the stories that people tell him about their companion animals. In hearing the owners' stories, he also learns about the owners themselves, thus leading the way for those of us who have an interest in the deep emotional significance of the companion animal relationship (Bradshaw 2011; Noonan 2008). The psychotherapist Boris Levenson, in the 1960s, was an important early influence in the field of Animal Assisted Therapies (AAT), focusing his research on children's psychological development and well-being (Levenson 1969; Franklin 1999; Vining 2003; Beck and Katcher 2003; Hines 2003; Walsh 2009a; 2002b; Favali and Milton 2010). Others followed, researching the effects of AAT and Animal Assisted Interventions (AAI) with various groups, such as the elderly, (Cusack and Smith 1984), children (Blue 1986), those with mental health problems (Corson and Corson 1980; Cusack 1988) and heart patients (Friedman et al. 1980).

Significant research into what is truly happening that is beneficial for humans in companion animal relationships, begins much later when veterinary science, in particular, attends to the human–animal bond. Hines (2003) gives a detailed historical account of how the term HAB developed in the 1970s growing firstly from veterinary research and attracting the attention of other professions across the world through conferences and publications. In tracing the growth of HAB, the multi-disciplinary, multi-national interest is apparent. The veterinarian, Bruce Fogle, took a positive view of the therapeutic effects of pet ownership (Fogle 1981, 1983) with far-reaching influence (e.g. Serpell 1998, 1995; Hines 2003). Notable others draw together work within the field, such as Katcher and Beck (1983), Anderson et al., (1984) and Rowan (1988). From these, and similar studies, the concepts of the human–animal bond, and its positive manifestations, have spread to such an extent that it is not possible to explore more than a limited number here. I have chosen to consider the most prominent recent work from several different disciplines, not only for its content concerning the human–animal relationship, but also because of what the studies say about the value and shortcomings of different methodologies within the research.

The literature that is most relevant to my study, published over the last twenty years, falls broadly into three strands: i) those devoted to the therapeutic effects of the human–animal relationship; ii) those focused on the emotional and development aspects of pet ownership; and iii) those which explore theories concerning human–animal bond within our culture.

i) Therapeutic effects: A great number of peer reviewed papers and books explore the therapeutic aspects of the relationship between humans and companion animals. The findings have influenced the development of AAT and AAI of many types. Odendaal (2002) used a scientific approach to exploring the benefits to people's mental health in his study of how human–dog interactions affect blood pressure and neurochemical changes which promote healing. An important outcome of Peacock et al.'s (2012) study of the connection between human–animal bonds and mental health, is to open up the discussion about the implications for mental health services. However, the results of these studies do not always support the expected beneficial outcomes for the target group. For example, when Phelps et al. (2008) investigated the effects of dogs' visits on depression, mood, and social interaction in elderly individuals living in a nursing home, they found that their empirical methodology proved inadequate. Although the residents said that they enjoyed the visits, the baseline assessment methods used in the study did not show sufficient evidence of beneficial effect without further research. However, Chur-Hansen et al. (2009) collected both quantitative and qualitative data for their study of companion animals and the impact they have on elderly women's physical and psychological health. They found that the data gave them enough evidence to support a finding that women with moderate attachment to their pets, experienced benefits which exceeded those experienced by women with low or high attachments. It seems that qualitative research has an important role to play in the field of health-based HAB and HAI research. The relevance to my study of the human–animal bond in everyday domestic settings, is that these studies support the theory that well-being accrues from the relationship. Such studies also colour modern thinking within our culture and thus influence attitudes to pet keeping and the companion animal relationship (e.g. Franklin 1999; Podberscek et al. 2000). It is also of interest to note the mixture of research methods used to make discoveries in the area, from the quantitative (Siegel 1990; Staats et al 2006) to mixed methodologies (Blue 1986; Wood et al. 2007; Chur-Hansen et al. 2009; Knight and Herzog 2009; Cavanaugh et al. 2008) and purely qualitative, such as Noonan (2008), Favali and Milton (2010) and Irvine (2013). Indeed, Favali and Milton (2010) use IPA to analyse the experiences of five disabled adults' experience of horse-riding. Their findings highlight the benefits to the participants' 'issues of trust, assertiveness and self-esteem' (p. 261). One of the reasons they chose a phenomenological approach for their study is that 'there is very little evidence of what people are actually experiencing when they are with animals' (p. 252). Gilbey et al. (2007) draw attention to the deficiency in quantitative methods within the field of HAB research in their study of the impact of companion animal ownership on loneliness. Unable to find evidence that loneliness is reduced in their sample, they suggest that their methods are restrictive, in that they 'fail to detect the qualitative changes that truly do occur' (p. 352).

ii) Emotional and developmental aspects: The areas of attachment, bereavement, child development and personal experiences of AAT find much attention. Influential studies include those of Noonan (2008), Robinson (1995), Beck and Katcher (1996), Stewart, et al., (1989) and Blue (1986). In addition, there are studies relating to the nature of dogs and cats, (Bradshaw 2011, 2013), and current studies on canine capacity for empathic response to humans (Coren 2012; Custance and Mayer 2012). Blue (1986) looks in detail at the child–pet relationship in the development of attachment and a range of developmental skills, both physical and psychological, in children. Her findings prompt her recommendations that the educational curriculum for young children should provide animal-related activities. Beck and Katcher (1996) consolidate a wealth of material, reinforcing their work on the emotional benefits of companion animal relationships. Stewart et al. (1989) focus on the complex nature of the loss of a companion animal and suggest that those in the caring professions, who are in contact with bereaved pet owners, should be 'particularly sensitive to the warning signs of depression, complicated bereavement, anxiety or panic states, suicidal thoughts and other affective disorders' (p. 157). Noonan's study (2008) is of direct relevance to Counsellors and Psychotherapists. Herself a Clinical Psychologist and Counsellor, she explores the significance of pets to their owners, drawing on 'psycho-analytical and attachment theory, ethology, veterinarians and literature' (p. 395) as well as her own personal experience of lingering grief after the death of her cat (p. 395). Unlike the majority of academics who study the human–animal bond, she confines her research to 'the everyday domestic tie between people and their pets' (p. 395), a perspective which matches that of my own study. Banning (2012), a Counsellor with a particular interest in promoting well-being in the workplace, experiences for herself the way in which horses facilitate therapy. She learns, through equine facilitated therapy (EFT), that 'if we listen, horses can teach us much about how we relate to the world and how we're experienced by others' (p. 18).

iii) Theories: There is also research that illuminates the theoretical landscape in which my topic is situated. Beck and Katcher's work (2003) addresses the two guiding theoretical influences on HAB research: namely biophilia hypothesis and social support theory. They argue that it is 'difficult to separate out biophilia, the cultural response to animals of different kinds ... and the effects of social support on both animals and humans'; and that both approaches need to be combined in order to avoid too 'narrow a focus on companion animals as the sole source of health benefits from the non-human environment' (p. 81). In simple terms, researchers should consider the impact of factors such as, the garden, countryside and birds when making claims that, for example, dog walking brings psychological benefits to people. Bradshaw (2011; 2013), in his anthrozoological studies of dogs and cats in human society, gives us new insights into their natures in order to promote a greater understanding of their roles as companion animals. While acknowledging the importance of the emotional bond, he is critical of people who attribute human characteristics to their dogs:

> Without an emotional bond, there would be no pets – and yet this bond can sometimes create problems for dogs and humans alike. The emotional bond between owner and the pet is often, perhaps to some degree always, bound up in anthropomorphic projections (Bradshaw 2011, p. 149).

In addition, he counters some of the present theories about the human–dog and human–cat relationships, and raises serious concerns about how the animals will fare as society changes. The sociologist, Adrian Franklin (1999), disagrees with Bradshaw's fear about the dangers of increasing anthropomorphism. Indeed, he sees anthropomorphism as widening the gap between humans and animals, the reverse of what he believes is occurring in modern society. He argues that as we grow to value animals as both therapeutic, and of ecological quintessence, the dangers of anthropomorphism are diminishing. His study examines changes in the British, Australian and North American social and cultural environments, and how the changes have impacted upon the ways we relate to animals and the natural world. When he considers the accumulated science concerning the health benefits of pet ownership, AAT and pet-facilitated therapy (PFT), he speculates that 'it may prove difficult to ignore their potential savings to burgeoning national health budgets' (p. 103). His positive views are compelling because they take into account both the scientific advances and the nature of our unique connection to animals. Serpell's (2002) perspective differs from Franklin's. He sees advantages in anthropomorphism believing that,

> Anthropomorphism has provided the opportunity to use animals as an alternative source of social support and the means to benefit emotionally and physically from this (Serpell 2002, p. 448).

These differing opinions on the values and dangers of attributing human feelings and motivations to animals each deserve consideration when hearing people's personal experiences. Podberscek et al.'s (2000) book brings together several important studies concerning the nature of the human–companion animal relationship. The book extends into an area which has been little-researched: how pet ownership is influenced by other current human relationships which might exist for the owners, and how pet ownership impacts on networks of family relationship: both important considerations for Counsellors (Walsh 2009b). Kobak (2009) seeks to define and measure the attachment bond, comparing it to the adult human attachment bond, and finding it has strong similarities. Knapp (1998) explores what lies behind the human–animal bond. She reaches into the historical evidence and the current developments in animal therapy, through her own personal experiences with dogs. Arguably the most influential study of human–animal relationships is Serpell (1998), first published in 1986, when studies in the field were first emerging, and since revised. He challenges us to explore the relationships more closely, both animal and human because,

> Pet-owners do not value their animals primarily as objects, but rather as subjects; as distinctive personalities with whom they have affectionate relationships not dissimilar to the kinds of affectionate relationships they have with close friends and relatives. If we wish to understand the possible contribution of pets to human health and welfare, then surely we should begin by exploring the influence of close relationships, in general, on our mental and physical condition (Serpell 1998, pp. 106–107).

While the human–animal relationship attracts attention widely across disciplines, it is nevertheless challenging to identify studies which truly focus on the everyday experience of pet owners. The ideas and directions within the material undoubtedly penetrate current attitudes surrounding pet ownership. However, it is striking that few studies look in-depth at the everyday experience of people sharing their homes, families, resources and time with pets. When Walsh (2009a) reviews the literature, she finds that 'the field of mental health has been slow to recognize the importance of these bonds in clinical theory, research and practice' (p. 462–463). Walsh discovers that 'attachments with companion animals have been undervalued and even pathologized in the field of mental health' (p. 462). The psychologist and psychotherapist, Owen (2008), reflects that the relationship that a client has with an animal is a significant part of the wider context of their lives, and thus deserves the attention of Counsellors: 'Consideration of a client's relationship with the animal world in isolation would seem limiting, but the exploration of this in relation to the overall context of their life seems to add an extra dimension of understanding' (p. 47).

My study aims to contribute to this 'extra dimension' through its focus on the everyday, domestic, non-deliberately therapeutic relationship which people have with their animals.

Participants

The following inclusion criteria were applied when selecting the sample:

- People who had experienced a meaningful, significant relationship with a companion animal for a period in their lives.
- For ethical reasons, people who had sufficient emotional support in the event of the interview bringing up troubling material for them.

The exclusion criteria for the sample were as follows:

- Again for ethical reason, people with whom I had a dual relationship, such as friendship or working relationship.
- Those who work with animals professionally such as farmers, zookeepers, animal welfare workers, zoologists, AAT or AAI specialists.

As I work as a Samaritan Volunteer Listener, I felt that the Samaritan organization could provide accessible and suitable participants. Although I intended to advertise for my participants, this proved unnecessary as my pilot interviewee referenced my first participant to me. The process of referencing continued, and thus I acquired a snowball sample (Denscombe 2014; Maykut and Morehouse 1994) consisting of two Samaritan volunteers and two Counsellors in training, each of whom met the inclusion criteria. The participants' profiles are as in Table 5. The participants selected their pseudonyms for the study; however, they each preferred that their animals' names remain unchanged.

	Anne	Violet	Louise	Charlotte
Age	Mid twenties	Early forties	Early forties	Early forties
Number of humans in household	Three: Anne, partner and sister	Two: Violet and daughter	Two: Louise and partner	One: Charlotte
Companion animal(s)	Two cats	Two cats	One dog	One horse, one foal, one dog, five cats
Profile	Samaritan volunteer	Samaritan volunteer	Counsellor in training	Counsellor in training

Table 5: Profiles of participants.

Data collection

Semi-structured interviews were planned. A series of questions and prompts were developed to encourage the participants to talk at length and in depth about their experiences (Smith et al. 2009). These questions were:

- Tell me about the pet that has been most significant to you (either past or present).
- Tell me about the ways your pet affects your mood.
- People speak of a bond – what is your feeling about that?
- What are your experiences of talking about your pet with other people?
- Is there anything else you'd like to add?

Findings

Although the participants each have their distinct characteristics, it has been possible to identify three master themes linking the data from each interview. The master themes have within them sub-themes that assist in capturing particular facets, qualities and details of the participants' experience (see Table 6):

Master Themes	Sub-themes
1: **Presence:** The everyday experience of wholeness within the home, and sensory pleasures.	1.1 Filling the spaces 1.2 Touch, sight, sound and play
2: **The Bond:** The experience of sharing, caring and understanding.	2.1 A constant witness 2.2 Extraordinary companionship 2.3 Understanding, reciprocity and caring
3: **Self and Enrichment:** The therapeutic experience.	3.1 Healing and Transformation 3.2 Connections and purpose 3.3: Identity and beliefs

Table 6: Master themes and sub-themes.

Master theme 1: Presence

Sub-theme 1.1: Filling the spaces: Violet says, *"I don't think a house is a home without an affectionate pet in it"*. The other participants, in their differing ways, echo her view. By filling the space with their physical presence, each of the animals provides stimuli to the senses that delight the participants. For Violet, the presence of her two young cats is intensely important. She had experienced a period without cats, owing to an allergy she developed. The allergy eventually disappeared and she introduced her present cats into the household. During the period without cats, *"the house was missing a wholeness"* that she felt acutely when her young daughter spent time away. She struggles to find words to express the power of her feelings: *"Going home to an empty house is just the most **awful** thing – I can't express – just, no, no other life in the house, no other being in the house – it just feels empty"*. Louise echoes the emptiness, and emphasizes that her dog's constant presence is hugely important and central to the space: *"I feel her presence ... there's a constant kind of sense of her there ... it's not that life revolves around, well maybe it does revolve around her, but I think her presence is very important in the house ... it's very odd, the house feels very empty without her in it. So I think she's got a very, a very positive presence"*. Louise experiences her dog, Joy, as filling not only the physical space of the house, but also an emotional space. It is an experience which is beyond her expectations: *"So I think that, how important she is really, and how, she does fill spaces physically but also emotionally. And that has been quite surprising"*. For Anne, her two cats' continual presence is important to her because she says, *"I didn't feel quite as alone"*. She speaks with pleasure of their pervasiveness, *"They're just usually there"*. One cat in particular: *"she's on my knee almost before I've managed to sit on the sofa, and she sleeps next to me in bed on the mattress and she's very much always there"*. Charlotte identifies her significant companion animal as her horse, Amber. Although they do not share a living space, Charlotte speaks of a time before having Amber when *"it was very lonely"*. She credits Amber with filling the lonely void. She also speculates that her house *"would feel empty"* without her dog and cats, which is not something she wants to experience.

Sub-theme 1.2: Touch, sight, sound and play: The consistent pleasure, both through the physical affection and humorous antics, is striking in Charlotte's account. Her five cats (Tom, Tabatha, Tennyson, Travis and Tilly) constantly entertain as *"they all have their own characters and they all do their own little thing"*. Moreover, they shower her with daily gifts: *"there's always something that one of them will bring to me each day, in terms of affection, or something that they do that can make me laugh"*. Violet returns several times to the visual pleasure her two cats (Lilith and Itse) bring. In her description she uses a striking metaphor expressing her admiration for their strength and beauty: *"They are like panthers, absolutely just gorgeous and sleek and beautiful"*. She speaks of their energy, personalities and of missing *"the contact ... the cuddling and playing"* if she is away from them. Anne uses the sensory words *"nuzzle"* and *"purr"* on four occasions to tell of the pleasure of touching and hearing her cats (Pepper and Kia). She admits, hesitantly, that their appearance triggers her maternal instinct: *"this is going to sound really weird – I think they are very good at looking cute – I find, I look at them – I think I get the same reaction to cats that most people get to babies, ... that they do something cute and you get that sort of, warm, sort of haarh"*. Louise describes her pleasure in her dog (Joy) as a delight in Joy's comic behaviour: *"if she is being told to do something she doesn't want to, there's a whole kind of grumbling that goes on – and if we say get off the sofa, she'll go, and instead of just sitting down, she'll do this whole turning around and around and around – sometimes for ages, making it known I think that she's not happy that she's not allowed to be on the sofa"*. Not only does Joy provide these comic mimes, but she also has a continual life-and-soul quality: *"she'll just go along with whatever's going on – as long as she's in the middle of it"*.

Master theme 2: The Bond: The experience of sharing, caring and understanding

Each participant feels strongly attached to her animals. They each speak of a reciprocal caring, and a sense that the animal knows them, sometimes in ways that are difficult to explain. For two participants in particular, the bond is particularly strong because their animals have been with them through significant periods of personal change and growth.

Sub-theme 2.1: A constant witness: Louise's dog has accompanied her as her only *"constant"* through the difficult journey after her marriage broke up eleven years ago: *"And that's the only thing in that time that has been constant, and I think about her that she and I have lived that **together**, even though she's obviously not experienced lots of the things that I've experienced. She's seen all of that – that's the idea of a witness – I really like that idea. Nobody else has been there through all of that, those things, and those changes"*. Charlotte also feels bonded with Amber because she has been with her through great difficulty: *"the last four or five years have been like a roller coaster – and she's been like the one constant who's always been there"*. That lasting companionship strengthened her to face the difficulties: *"it felt like it was us together and it didn't really matter what else was going on in my life"*. Violet expressed fierce commitment to keeping Lilith and Itse with her: *"There is just no way I could have not had those cats in my life – my best friends"*, despite taking risks and overcoming obstacles in her rented home where animals are prohibited. Anne laughed as she describes the ways in which Pepper and Kia follow her every move, like it or not, *"... They're just always, yeah, there're always there. You're trying to shoo them off if I need to get up or anything else, it's a nightmare because as soon as I move them they are trying to get back"*.

Sub-theme 2.2: Extraordinary companionship: Anne valued her relationship with Pepper and Kia because she is their special human: *"I am the person they come to. They are very much my cats – even though there's other people, they will always have a preference for me over anybody else"*. Their preference for her makes their bond clan-like: *"It's almost like a little pack, like a little unit"*. There is also a sense of exclusiveness in Violet's strong description of her relationship with Lilith and Itse in which she reiterates *"my"* and *"mine"*: *"they are **my** cats, they are not **mine** and my partner's cats, not **mine** and my mum and dad's cats, they're **my** cats and I've raised them since they were kittens – and I think, the bond's stronger there"*. Louise also feels that she and Joy *"have a more important bond"* than the dog has with anyone else. Whilst she queries the notion, nevertheless it is real to her: *"... although she's happy with other people – and I might be imagining this ... I do think there is a bond here"*. The dread she has of losing Joy indicates the strength of the attachment: *"I've been thinking, because she's getting grey and everything, how am I going to manage when she's gone"*. Charlotte struggled to find adequate words to express the *"really special bond"* she feels with her horse Amber: *"It's just been a really special bond that - it's kind of hard to put into words ... it's almost like we understood each other"*. When she says, *"she's always been where I've turned to I suppose the most for support"*, she reveals the depth and magnitude of the relationship.

Sub-theme 2.3: Understanding, reciprocity and caring: In turning to Amber for 'support', Charlotte felt understood and nurtured. They worked through their problems in unison with each able to progress no faster than the other, and a sense that Amber was reflecting Charlotte's unresolved issues: *"we hadn't worked through all her* (Amber's) *problems, mainly because they were probably coming from me, and I haven't worked through my own problems"*. Louise experienced 'trust' between herself and Joy as an important reciprocal bond at a time when she felt betrayed. The memory is painful, and she hesitates before committing to the word 'trust': *"I could give her I guess as well, (sounding tearful) a fanciful word to use, trust that she had in me to care for her, and that was nice because I was very devastated. But she kind of helped me to … put myself together again I think. She was very much part of that process of … yeah, re-building myself I suppose … I think it was hard for me to trust people, but it wasn't hard for me to trust my dog. I just trust her, she's loyal – she's there and she's not going anywhere. And she won't let me down"*. Louise receives from Joy a mirroring of the loyalty and trust she gives. Violet feels that her cats cared in an intriguingly intuitive way when she was pregnant: *"… before I knew I was pregnant, they were both on my stomach, and as I got bigger they kind of draped over the bump and – they were looking after me and the baby"*. She speaks of having a *"purr or a random conversation while I make a cup of tea in the morning"*, and of being greeted when she comes through the door, with a powerful sense of her cats interacting and understanding her. Similarly, Anne speculates that there could be *"a protective bond"* with her cats. Kia, in particular *"picks up on things"* and she gives an example concerning her sister's panic attacks: *"… if she has a panic attack, she'll find a cat on her knee, which is really weird. …. sort of intuitive emotional – they don't necessarily understand what's going on but that pain or comfort"*. Her description conveys her difficulty in making sense of her experience along with a conviction that the cats have an understanding of some sort, which informs their caring behaviour.

Master theme 3: Self and Enrichment: The therapeutic experience

Each participant has their own story of the benefits their animals have brought to their lives. These benefits include helping to restore emotional well-being and encouraging social engagement. The sense of purpose is apparent in each account, rooted in the routines and responsibilities their animals bring into their lives.

Sub-theme 3.1: Healing and transformation: Louise made a conscious decision to acquire a dog while suffering the emotional pain of her marriage breakdown, and not just any dog. She says, *"I thought that the best way to get some happiness back in my life was to buy a dog. ... I don't know what had got into my head but what I thought I really want to buy is a cocker spaniel, and I want to call her Joy"*. She is tearful as she describes how she *"didn't feel like interacting with people"*. Joy shielded her from having to engage with others before she felt ready: *"I didn't want to socialize so I'd be able to say at work, oh I can't come out because I've got to go home and feed the dog. I'm sure people thought I was a bit mad, but that's fine. It just gave me an excuse not to interact with people till I really wanted to on a social level – it was really useful"*. Beyond simply shielding her, Joy gave her *"optimism"* and a *"focus of enjoyment"* at a time when she *"might have been a lot more miserable"*. Louise says, *"she really picked me up at a time when I was pretty low"*. Joy was *"something to hold on to that was good ... And it worked, yeah it worked"*. Her dog eased her back into the world without demanding much in return: *"... she gave me some stability – looking after her, taking her out, routine, some sort of interaction that didn't expect anything of me except very basic kind of actions"*. Charlotte's story emphasizes the transformation she experienced through her relationship with Amber, her horse. *"It's hard to explain how I used to feel when I first had her – I felt I couldn't really express myself to anyone. I felt very isolated in a lot of ways. I felt I couldn't really talk to anyone in many ways. And yet when I was with her I felt that everything was alright ... Yeah, (Slowly, thoughtfully) I don't think I would be where I am – she got me through a lot ... just* in terms of giving me that kind of reflection, that ... horses whatever you do they give you a very honest reflection of your emotions and what you are doing – which I suppose is a bit like Person-Centred". Violet, too, believes Pepper and Kia played a significant part in her recovery from mental ill-health: "They do lift my mood ... they've been part of my recovery really because I had – over the three years – I've had a couple of breakdowns, ended up on medication – and it wasn't until I got the kittens last year that I actually suddenly started feeling a hell of a lot better". Anne also speaks of a therapeutic benefit she experiences from her cats: "I've always had problems with depression, anxiety ... and I got them at a point I was feeling quite down – and I think they just – yeah, the things they do – the little quirks just made me smile. So, I think having them around always made me happier".

Sub-theme 3.2: Connections and purpose: Furthermore, Anne's cats give her a reason to keep going which she recognizes as valuable: "It gives me another reason, if you like, to keep going, and, to do that next day when I don't want to do that next day". The responsibility Anne feels for Pepper and Kia adds to their motivating effect. "... we adopted them, and we adopted them to look after them for the rest of their lives, ... we have a duty to provide them with food and shelter, comfort and everything else. ... For me it gives a sense of purpose ... I have someone, something that's dependent on me". She uses the pronoun "someone", revealing their person-like significance to her. Violet too experiences her cats as motivating her to recover when she is emotionally debilitated and to keep going for their sakes: "... if it hadn't have been for them I wouldn't have had a reason to not – to push myself to normalisation and sort myself out so they do have a massive effect on my mood". And similar to Anne, Violet surprises herself when she refers to them as if human in her description of their motivating effect: "I think my recovery was a lot quicker ... it was somebody else, 'somebody' *else* [tone of querying her expression 'somebody'] *I had to function for"*. The sense of *"huge responsibility"* also features in Charlotte's account. Strikingly, she is clear that the way her cats' behaviour changed towards her taught her about how she related to people and animals during her troubled time: *"... as I gradually came out of myself I noticed the change in them, that they wanted to spend time with me and were a lot more playful, so I think they taught me a lot about myself and how I could come across to people and to animals"*. Louise feels it was important to her that Joy helped her engage with others at a level which felt pleasurable and undemanding while she was recovering: *"I could engage with other dog-walkers and I had a nice little group of people I'd meet most mornings – we'd chat about our dogs and that's all we did, we didn't go into anything else about who we were – and I found that level of engagement sufficient at that time"*. Now that she has come through the difficult period, she still derives pleasure from the social connections and appreciation which Joy brings: *"People will stop you and tell you the whole story about rescuing their dog and – I like that, that sort of engagement. And I like people liking her and giving her a fuss, – at the corner shop, every time we go they give her lots of treats"*.

Sub-theme 3.3: Identity and beliefs: Louise is habitually open about how important her dog is in her life; her commitment to Joy is part of her identity. *"I've been **very** open about how important my dog is in helping my emotional well-being and my mental health at kind of key moments"*. During the early period when she was very low, she adjusted her working hours in order to incorporate Joy into her life, and reaped benefits: *"I just negotiated my working hours to fit around looking after her ... I kind of built my life around looking after her – and that kind of, took me off, distracted me from other stuff that was difficult"*. Joy's importance to her is reflected in her belief that others are missing out, *"poor them"*: *"if you haven't got that, if* *you haven't had that experience then you don't understand how significant a pet can be"*. Violet echoes Louise's belief: *"I find it quite difficult to form a bond sometimes with people who are completely anti-pets – it's like, how can you not have anything in your life?"* In early childhood, Violet felt a sense of belonging and being needed when she formed a bond with the family cat. Her place in the family was enhanced along with her self-worth: *"I felt special, because ... my little brother was more favoured, by my parents ... and, the cat, the cat was mine, made me happy ... gave me a bit more belonging, or needed, wanted"*. Violet identifies strongly with cats as a species declaring her affinity cheerfully to the world. She has her own website with a feline name, and wears a tee-shirt with *"... two little eyes, and it just says 'feral' across it. ... people know I'm the crazy cat lady"*. Similarly, Anne is happy to incorporate cats firmly into her identity: *"I'm probably you know one of these people who's most likely to be voted crazy cat lady by everybody that I know"*. In her workplace, Anne has chosen to decorate her identity badge with cats, partly to personalize her appearance in an environment where people wear uniforms: *"like a load of Stepford wives – so I suppose that's my, my personalisation"*. She also feels that the images cheer others, particularly as children visit her department: *"I think cats generally – they make you smile ... you think about something like that, and it makes you smile, then it makes your day a bit brighter"*. Charlotte believes that her affinity with animals relates to her childhood experience of being adopted: *"a person who's adopted as a child quite often will put a lot of our relationships in with animals"*. She notices that she bonds easily with animals: *"There was just something about me bonding with animals"*. Animals seem to arrive without her seeking them: *"a lot of these animals I wasn't really looking for them, they just happened to come into my life"*. Her relationship with Amber is such an important part of her self-concept that she feels conflicted when her boyfriend spends time with Amber, and through his voluntary work, takes disabled people to see her: *"I felt a bit jealous at first – and then I felt a bit guilty, why should I keep her to myself"*. Though acknowledging these feelings, and growing in self-awareness, Charlotte has developed an interest in equine facilitated therapy (EFT), a direction she is now considering for her future career. In learning to share Amber, she has made her horse a yet more central part of her life.

Through linking the four participants' testimonies across the master and sub-themes, commonalities and idio-syncrasies have been exposed. Taken together, the positive, life-enhancing aspects of the companion relation-ships are expressed in the array of received pleasures: laughter, fun, happiness, delight, joy, warmth, generosity, understanding, wholeness, wonder and affirmation. These pleasures are felt to be reliable, uncomplicated, healing and transforming.

Discussion

The words of the four participants give vivid testimony to the value of the animal companions in their lives. The essence of their experiences has been captured within three master themes. The sense of not being alone, which emerges as important to each of the participants, is explored in a number of the studies. No matter where other family members might be, the presence of the animal is a comforting constant (Cavanaugh et al 2008; Staats et al. 2006; Sable 2013; Wood et al. 2007). Louise does not have to see her dog to have a *"constant"* sense of her *"positive presence"*. Each of the participants valued the sense of presence their animals give within their homes. They express a dread of the emptiness they would experience without them. Violet speaks of her house *"missing a wholeness"* which Walsh (2009a) believes is a fundamental part of the bond with companion animals: 'Bonds with companion animals may not be our whole lives, but they can make our lives whole' (p. 476). Stewart et al. (1989), when considering bereavement following the loss of a companion animal, tells of the emptiness pet owners can suffer, once their home is no longer shared with the animal. Research shows that companion animals can shield owners against this emptiness (Chur-Hansen et al. 2009; Franklin 1999; Siegel 1990). It is the participants' expectation that their animals will provide this shield. Franklin (1999) looks at the changes in modern western society that have contributed to the acceptance of companion animals as a welcome buffer against loneliness: 'pets can provide companionship, love and attention to humans wherever it is required. In late modernity we are now self-consciously aware of their value and unselfconscious in acknowledging it' (p. 104). The impact of the social context which Franklin describes is evident in the participants' expectations of their pets.

It is not simply a passive role that the animals play in filling the home; the playfulness and the sensory pleasures bring real benefits (Beck and Katcher 1996; Noonan 2008; Owen 2008; Robinson 1995; Sable 2013). According to Beck and Katcher (1996), companion animals affect us in primarily visual ways, tapping into our hidden wishes to behave badly, idiotically and clownishly:

> ... the dog can be thought of as a mime, a comic psychotherapist who represents to us in pictures the content of our unconscious urges and the contradictions between those urges and our civilized way of life, a function performed by traditional clowns (p. 183).

Indeed the participants echo this joy in their animals' cheeky, cute, clever and quirky qualities: laughter is a major part of the relationships. Louise delights in the comic mime her dog, Joy, performs when told to get off the sofa. Cat owners, Anne, Charlotte and Violet, each tell of the daily pleasures of watching their cats in action. When Violet likens her cats to panthers, she is admiring their sleekness and beauty, making a link to wildness and danger, which Beck and Katcher (1996) recognize as part of the human–animal bond. Anne describes herself as *"not a particularly maternal person"*, yet she feels her response to her cats is a *"different expression"* of the maternal instinct. Serpell (1995) writes of how 'humans have exaggerated or enhanced the neotenous, child-like qualities of companion animals through generation of unconscious selection' (p. 143). Rather than denigrating the neoteny and anthropomorphizing of pets, he believes that 'by virtue of their resemblance to children, pets can undoubtedly provide their owners with comparable psychological rewards' (Serpell 1995, p. 143). The sheer fascination and delight which Violet takes in her cats' appearance is reflected in Knapp's description of her dog:

> I have become enchanted by the small asymmetrical whorls of white fur on either side of her chest ... by her eyes, which are watchful and intelligent, the color of chestnuts ... I seem to spend a great deal of time just staring at the dog, struck by how mysterious and beautiful she is to me (Knapp 1998, p. 6).

The rewards of cuddling, stroking and hearing the purr of a cat, feature strongly in the three cat-owning participants' accounts. We know from several studies that these aspects bring benefits to physical and mental well-being (e.g. Robinson 1995). Because we can touch our animals and receive their nuzzlings and licks, this gives the relationship a particular quality which is necessarily missing in the relationship between client and Counsellor. Beck and Katcher tell us that 'the difficult art in therapy is achieving a mutual feeling of intimacy without touching' (1996, p. 92). They are not saying that dogs make better psychotherapists than humans, but they are struck by the power of their physical intimacy in bestowing well-being. Developments in AAT and AAI rely on there being a strong bond between people and companion animal relationship, so that the animal can be brought into a person's life specifically to give therapeutic or practical aid. The positive developments in these fields of research can be seen to have had an impact on the participants' experiences. Louise reveals that her belief in the benefits of people's relationships with companion animals has coloured her thoughts and intentions. She is unequivocal that she expected her dog to be *"the best way"* to bring happiness back into her life. With a clear image of her spaniel prior to finding her, Louise names her 'Joy': a significant naming which expressed an expectation (Noonan 2008). The names that people give their pets are frequently a 'word or symbol that links the animal and the person' (Beck and Katcher 1996, p. 14); Louise's bond with Joy and the dog's identity existed before they became a reality. The expectation alone might bring benefits and resilience (Staats et al. 2006; Wells 2011). Charlotte's belief in her horse's therapeutic qualities gave her a desire to share her with others in need, and she envisages a future for herself in EFT. She, too, is strongly influenced by her belief in the companion animal bond as bringing benefits. That the bond exists is widely accepted and exploited in AAT and AAI; the nature of the bond is scrutinized and compared to human attachment theories. Sable (2013) is clear that the bond has significant attributes of an adult attachment as defined by Bowlby (1973; 1980):

> A threat to the figure's accessibility will evoke protest and other measures to ward off separation or loss, and a permanent loss will evoke grief and mourning. Once we understand these aspects of attachment, the devotion to pets begins to make sense. Our pets ... provide proximity, and prompt positive feelings such as joy and laughter that make people feel less alone and lonely; in other words they furnish a component of attachment that promotes well-being and security, as well as affording opportunities for caregiving and commitment (Sable 2013, p. 98).

She identifies much that is similar to that of an adult human attachment, though with an emphasis on the care-giving and commitment elements of the attachment. In his work, defining and measuring the attachment bonds between people and their dogs, Kobak (2009) discusses Kurdek's (2009) findings, and he also concludes that the bond is more consistent with that of caregiver than a true attachment figure, since the relationship does not entirely fulfil all the criteria, such as 'safe haven' and 'secure base behaviour', as defined by Ainsworth (1991) and Bowlby (1980). Nevertheless, he is clear that there is a case for further research to establish if the affectional bond goes deep enough for a dog to be a true attachment figure. Stewart et al. (1989) believe that, '... it is the pet's preverbal attachment attitude that satisfies the human repressed need for nurturance. The pet's nonverbal acceptance and response to the human enables trust' (p. 149). That ability to communicate non-verbally, and to elicit a caring response, certainly contributes to the participants' sense of being needed and appreciated. Yet each participant also attests to a specialness in the relationship. Knapp (1998) finds the attachment to have an extraordinary type of closeness, a 'brand of proximity' that is not one she would want to have with another human being; to be 'that inseparable or entwined' (p. 226) would be intolerable. Charlotte's bond with Amber relies strongly on her care-giving: *"I think just me taking my time helped her and she's come and helped me. So, it's a very special relationship"*. Anne is so committed to caring for her cats, that she believes finding a house to rent which is suitable for the animals is more important than finding suitable accommodation for herself. She could live anywhere, but the cats depend on her to provide the right type of home for them. Violet feels duty-bound to care when she defies the landlord's regulations in order to provide a home for her cats. And Louise alters her working life in order to fit in with her puppy's care needs. The lived-experience of the participants is certainly testament to the 'sense of being truly entwined' (Knapp 1998, p. 226).

Walsh (2009b) cites Allen's (1995) work on coping mechanisms, which found that 'confiding in pets to "discuss" difficult life situations greatly relieved stress' (p. 483). This is borne out in Charlotte's sense that Amber eased her through the difficult times, and by sharing her trouble with her horse, she was strengthened: *"it felt like it was us together"*. Violet speaks of her pleasure in the *"random conversations"* she has with her cats. Banning (2012) tells of the empathetic qualities of horses she encounters in EFT, chiming with Charlotte's sense that her horse understands her and reflects her emotions in a manner that enables her to understand herself better. To her, it feels like 'Person-Centred' empathy, even though it is inconceivable that an animal could achieve empathic understanding which requires a 'capacity to track and sense accurately the feelings and personal meanings' of the person (Mearns and Thorne 2013, p. 15). Nevertheless, the participants each experience something akin to empathic understanding. The nature of animals' understanding of humans has attracted much research, particularly concerning dogs and humans (e.g. Bradshaw 2011; Fogle 1983, 1981; Knapp 1998; Serpell 1995, 1998). Beck and Katcher (1996) make a direct comparison between dogs and Person-Centred therapists:

> A Rogerian analyst is not unlike a Labrador retriever. The Labrador retriever is certainly not directive. He gives no advice ... He is perceived as empathetic (p. 92).

Bradshaw's (2011) extensive study of dogs, led him to conclude that although their emotional lives are more limited than those of humans, nevertheless 'dogs share our capacity to feel joy, love, anger, fear and anxiety' (p. 210). They also read human body language with acute accuracy. The debates and research continue as to the capacity for empathy in dogs (e.g. Coren 2012; Custance and Mayer 2012). However, the lived-experience of the participants is that their animals understand them in some way, which gives them a positive feeling of well-being.

In Irvine's (2013) ethnographical study, the narratives of homeless people provide powerful evidence of animal-companionship as 'Lifesavers and Lifechangers'. Louise hesitates and backtracks when she uses the same word 'lifesaver': "... *life-saver would be a very dramatic way of putting it – in some ways I suppose* – [pause, tearful voice] – *yes*". However, it is in her mind that Joy played a redemptive role in her life. By providing consistent, reliable bonds, companion-animals have the power to 'facilitate transitions through disruptive life changes' (Walsh 2009a, p. 470). Each of the participants attests in her own way to this restorative power: Louise through her marriage breakup; Charlotte through her period of anguish and withdrawal; Anne through her depression and anxiety; and Violet through her periods of mental ill-health. During these periods of difficulty, the participants appreciated the ways in which their animals helped in restoring their well-being. Violet and Anne both feel that their cats began the process of lifting their low mood during periods of depression. The companion animal bond's positive effect on stress, depression and anxiety finds support in many research studies (e.g. Anderson et al. 1984; Robinson 1995; Rowan 1988; Siegel 1990). During her recovery, Louise's dog shielded her from the demands of social interactions for which she felt unready, as well as facilitating an easy level of social interaction with other dog-walkers: *"There wasn't any kind of deep level of interaction or any expectation, it was just ... nice to just talk about inconsequential things that dogs had been doing"*. This undemanding communication with others is seen as significantly beneficial in many studies (e.g. Irvine 2013; Robinson 1995; Serpell 1995, 1998; Wood et al. 2007). Indeed Wood et al. (2007) detect a 'social lubricant effect of pets', particularly dogs, because they entice their owners outdoors into their neighbourhoods. Charlotte's horse, Amber, helped her to break free from her isolation and inability to express her herself, through an emotional connection that she compares to the Person-Centred Counselling Approach. Amber gave her *"a very honest reflection"* of her emotions, something which Knapp (1998) attests to in her study of the connections between human beings and animals. Owen (2008) notices that her counselling clients

> ... who report intense difficulties relating to human beings sometimes describe very positive relations with their pets or horses. They often cite the consistency and unconditional nature of their animal's affection as the reason. It is true that animals do not judge a human being

111

by their intelligence, achievements, status or attractiveness and this perhaps alleviates some of the pressures in human to human interactions (p. 49).

Charlotte's experience with Amber echoes Owen's observations. Her troubled history left her wary of close human relationships. However, she trusts horses to let her try and fail: *"What I have found over the years is that animals are the most forgiving creatures. It doesn't matter if you get something wrong – you can try again – they'll deal with it"*. The easiness and reliability of the relationships, seems to alleviate stress for the participants. During her divorce, Louise welcomed the positive contrast of relating to her dog as opposed to dealing with the complexity of human relationships. Beck and Katcher (1996) emphasize the constancy of animals' responses to their owners as an important factor in conferring a sense of being safe and wanted: 'A pet's welcome is restorative and signals that everything is as it was when you left; everything is safe, and you have not changed, either' (p. 29). The sense of being 'greeted' is important to the participants. As Lorenz (2002) says, it is impossible to feel alone if at least one being is pleased to see you. Enthusiastic greeting is not the only aspect of the animals' behaviour that is affirming and a boost to self-esteem. The feeling of being the special one in the animal's life confers self-worth. There is evidence in each of the participants' accounts that their animals are motivating in ways that are life-enhancing. The benefits to people's physical health (e.g. Cavanaugh et al. 2008; Friedmann et al. 1980; Siegel 1993) through pet ownership depend heavily upon the motivational aspects of the relationship with the animal, as do the psychological benefits (Fawcett and Gullone 2001; Fogle 1981, 1983; Knight and Herzog 2009; Levenson 1969; Odendaal 2002; Peacock et al. 2012). In the context of recovery from illness, Noonan (2008) remarks on how people will often 'do something for their pet that they would not do for themselves, and this enhances their sense of being needed' (p. 404), thus speeding up their recovery. Violet endorses this benefit in her account of recovering quickly from a panic attack because the cats needed her: *"they actually really helped me pull through that … I could have quite easily been in a state for several hours"*. It is not only during difficult times that the companion animals supply a central importance in the participants' lives. The animals are bound up in their companion human's identity. Charlotte recognises, in herself, a drive towards being with animals. She also notices that she attracts animals to her. She speculates that having been adopted and troubled in childhood might have increased the intensity of the bond with animals, a view which Walsh (2009a) supports through her experience of counselling clients. Both Anne and Violet embrace cats into their identities, and Louise is adamant that others *"are really missing out on something really special"* if they have not experienced how special the relationship can be. She feels *"blessed"*. Harraway (2003) appears to be in tune with Anne, Louise, Charlotte and Violet, when she says that humans are also companion animals: 'There cannot be just one companion species; there have to be at least two to make one. It is in the syntax; it is in the flesh' (p. 12); and their strong bonds and connections with their animals are special, deep and important enough for each participant to trumpet them to the world.

Indeed the participants are enthusiastic and open in exploring the bonds they feel. There are few moments when they hesitate or trivialize. Yet these moments occur noticeably when they speak with a degree of anthropomorphism that causes them discomfort. It seems that cultural influences on their feelings about anthropomorphism might spring from negative views such as those of Bradshaw (2011), rather than the more positive views of Franklin (1999) and Serpell (2002). However, the data are insufficient to support the notion that people might be reluctant to share their deep feelings about their companion animals.

Conclusion

There are constraints and limitations that affect the research. It is a small-scale study thus limiting the data to that collected from four individuals. From such a small, homogeneous sample, it is not possible to arrive at generalizations. Further, phenomenological analysis relies on the interpretation of the participants' use of language (Willig 2008). Indeed, it can be argued that the complexity of language itself, as used by participants, is beyond the analytical scope of the IPA method. Language constrains, shapes or prescribes meaning (Willig 2008); hence, McLeod (2011) cautions researchers to take a tentative approach to drawing conclusions from the data. Spinelli (2005) speaks of phenomenological research as 'exhaustive, time-consuming, fraught with interpretative dangers, and never complete' (p. 137), and these features certainly impact upon this study. However, he also highlights the 'depth of value and meaning to all participants that traditional research never begins to reach' (p. 137); a balance of difficulty and reward that I have embraced.

I chose the subject for this study because my personal experience led me to suspect that the day-to-day, taken-for-granted experience of the companion animal relationship was life-enhancing. The narratives of Anne, Charlotte, Louise and Violet lend strong support to my originating premise. In the main, the literature in the area also chimes with my findings, particularly that of therapists Banning, Owen, Walsh and Noonan. I share similar experiences to those of Owen (2008).

She noticed one day that when her anxious client focused on a blue tit outside during a counselling session, he became 'instantly calmer' (p. 47). When one of my clients spotted a fox through the window during a session, he suddenly relaxed, laughed and consequently our rapport grew. Another client, anxious over grave troubles in her life, smiled and grew calm as she spoke of her dog, an oasis of joy in her distress. Moreover, I remember callers to Samaritans who spoke of their pets as an anchor, helping them contain suicidal ideations; this is a phenomenon that Walsh (2009a) has also experienced in her work with clients. As a result of hearing the testaments of my participants, I feel increasingly able to recognize the importance of the human–animal bonds in my clients' lives.

There is nothing peripheral or trivial about the relationships the participants describe with their companion animals. Indeed the centrality and importance in their lives is striking. Yet, the participants' stories go beyond what I expected. It was unexpected that each would reveal that they had emerged from difficult times in their lives with a sense that their companion animal relationship had been res-torative, sustaining and motivating. The companionship of animals is, of course, not a ubiquitous panacea; indeed many people are uncomfortable near animals. Animals, wild or domesticated, have an array of negative aspects which humans can encounter, such as allergies, phobias, nuisance, disease and physical danger (Bradshaw 2013, 2011; Franklin 1999; Owen 2008; Podberscek et al. 2000). Nevertheless, the benefits to well-being are indisputable, and supported in the lived-experiences of the participants. Owen (2008) writes that:

> In the course of therapy, the client may spontaneously describe their interactions with animals or other aspects of

the natural world. In doing so they perhaps provide a wealth of information about their beliefs, values and the processes in which they engage. Consideration of a client's relationship with the animal world in isolation would seem limiting but the exploration of this in relation to the overall context of their life seems to add an extra dimension of understanding (p. 51).

It is the 'extra dimension of understanding' that the findings of this study endorse. As a Person-Centred Counsellor, I find it salutary to consider that, for some people, there might be times when the transforming qualities of empathy, unconditional positive regard and congruence are more readily assessable through their animal relationship. Sheldrake (2000) notices the power of the animal's unconditional love:

For clients with low self-esteem, it is difficult to accept that any human can have much regard for them, and so it is hard to feel counsellors really accept them ... they feel that if all were revealed, the acceptance would be withdrawn. By contrast, they can easily believe that their animal loves them unconditionally (p. 80).

In Sheldrake's description, the animal is more of a substitute for the therapist than an ally in the therapy. At times, the four participants experienced this extreme when their animals gave them what no human could. It seems that for some, the fur-coated companion can fit their emotional needs, offering a uniquely valuable relationship when life feels dark. And, in the main, it is not a relationship that the participants are hesitant to discuss, nor do they trivialize their experiences. When I embarked upon this study, I suspected that people might feel inhibited in speaking about the depth of the bond; such a finding could be a useful factor for Counsellors to consider when working with clients. Little emerged to support this notion, thus further research would be needed in order to establish if such a phenomenon is prevalent. With my small, purposive sample of four, it was not possible to explore this aspect. However, it might be fruitful to interview experienced Counsellors who have worked with clients who have significant companion animal bonds, to continue the investigation. In the field of mental health, Walsh (2009a) is clear that research and training pay scant attention to the human–animal bond. She believes that: '… we can enrich clinical practice through a more holistic and open-minded view of the potential contribution of animal bonds to human healing and well-being' (p. 476). Following this study, I con-cur with her, as it has confirmed the important contribution of pets to the participants' happiness and well-being. To prize the precious bonds that clients might have with their animals, adds a significant dimension to our understanding of their world. As such, I suggest that the human–animal bond merits attention in counselling training, research and practice. It is appropriate to give Louise the final words as she summarizes the well-being she experiences: *"all the pressures of life, there's something easy and simple about my dog and the relationship I have with her. And that's great – I think that's great"*.

CHAPTER FOUR

NON-PHYSICAL ABUSE OF WOMEN WITHIN INTIMATE HETEROSEXUAL RELATIONSHIPS

Christine Hurst

Introduction

This chapter aims to provide an understanding of non-physical abuse (NPA), which occurs within the context of an intimate heterosexual relationship when there is no physical abuse (PA). It explores the experience of female Counsellors for two reasons; one, they are likely to have access to supervision and personal counselling in the event of painful issues being touched upon; and two, personal development training, a requirement of Counsellor training, will aid the recognition of NPA as it is often misunderstood, unrecognized and unseen.

NPA can be experienced with, or without, domestic violence, with most research being done in the context of violent relationships. This is in spite of the fact that, according to the British Crime Survey, of the 6% of women who were victims of domestic abuse, 57% suffered emotional abuse (EA) compared to 27% who sustained physical injuries (Hoyle 2013). The most salient feature of emotional abuse is its insidious nature (Outlaw 2009; Lachkar 2000; Lammers et al. 2005), with many types of emotionally abusive behaviour appearing socially acceptable (Lammers et al. 2005). Evans (1993) believes that the oppression of verbal abuse is so deeply woven into the fabric of society that it often goes unnoticed. Outlaw (2009) identifies four major types of NPA: emotional, psychological, economic and social abuse. However, the presence of one form of NPA does not mean that all types are present. Women can experience NPA for years without recognizing their partner's behaviour as abusive (Carlyle et al. 2008; O'Hagan 2006, 1995; Zink et al. 2003; Miller 1995). NPA is less identifiable than PA with a resultant unseen population (Carlyle et al. 2008). As there are no visible wounds (Miller 1995), the media cannot frame NPA as physical, thereby obscuring the impact and the resulting pain, and so make it doubly invisible (Sims 2008). Victims often wish that the abuser would hit them so they would have concrete proof of abuse, or a perceived justifiable excuse to leave the relationship (Dueckman 2012). Not recognizing the abuse can negatively affect victims' ability to defend against and recover from it (Marshall 1996). Women often report that forms of non-physical abuse have a more devastating effect on them than any physical injury (Outlaw 2009; Seff et al. 2008; Ro and Lawrence 2007; Bancroft 2002; Loring 1994). The effects of NPA can be emotional loneliness, despair, guilt, confusion, fear and anger, feelings of not being good enough, a sense of failure, diminished self-esteem and identity (Lammers et al. 2005).

This qualitative study was undertaken so that the lived-experience of women who had experienced NPA within an intimate relationship, when there was no PA, could be explored. The aim of the study was to expand the research on NPA when experienced by women in an intimate heterosexual relationship, when there is no PA. This research explores: the nature and effects of NPA; how and when it was recognized; any positive or negative coping skills used; the awareness of NPA of those experiencing it and others who may see it; if the relationship continued or ended and why; and what made participants vulnerable to being abused. The research aims to increase Counsellors' awareness of NPA in order to inform their work with a vulnerable population, as Counsellors can dismiss, or overlook, NPA when there is no overt conflict or physical assault (James and Mackinnon 2010).

I decided to research NPA as it is meaningful to me, due to my experience of NPA within an intimate relationship. On researching the literature available about NPA, it was found that most research was linked with physical or sexual abuse (Lammers et al. 2005), rather than being studied as behaviour in its own right. As this study researches NPA when there is no PA, I believe it will be a valuable addition to existing literature. My interest in this subject stems from being a child of the 1950s when men were the head of the household and expected to keep 'their women' in line; with women expected to defer to them. My views about life in my teenage years, twenties, and thirties, were formed from growing up in a patriarchal society. I took many of my expectations and relationship 'rules' for granted and without question. It was not until much later in life that I appreciated how much of my power I had given away. In my own life, and that of friends and family, I often see and experience instances of controlling and unpleasant behaviour, and have questioned when this becomes abuse as many types of emotionally abusive behaviour can appear socially acceptable (Lammers et al. 2005). My work in women's centres in the North West has exposed me to clients who have experienced NPA, and it seems surprising to me that violence and abuse towards women was not discussed publicly until the 1970s (Miller 2006). Working in the Counselling profession, I am aware of the insidious nature of NPA (Lachkar 2000; Lammers et al. 2005) and how difficult it can be to spot, especially as victims often don't consider themselves to be abused (Carlyle et al. 2008; O'Hagan 2006, 1995; Zink et al. 2003; Miller 1995). In fact, women may believe it is they who are at fault (Sims 2008). It is this unrecognized, and unseen, aspect to NPA that has inspired this research with the aim of helping NPA to become recognized and seen.

What the literature says

Researchers, such as McGee and Wolfe (1991) have struggled to define emotional abuse. Even the terms 'emotional' and 'psychological', used to label NPA, are often used interchangeably (James and MacKinnon 2010; O'Hagan 1995). It is this lack of agreement that makes it difficult to compare research findings (Lammers et al. 2005). So although awareness of emotional abuse has been rising (Loring 1994), until recently, research has been comparatively stagnant with discussions limited to defining terminology (Sorsoli 2004; Follingstad 2007; Ro and Lawrence 2007). Lack of research into 'pure' emotional abuse has also been hampered as it is generally, inextricably linked with physical or sexual abuse in existing literature (Lammers et al. 2005). Lammers et al. define emotional abuse as:

> The patterned non-physical degradation of one person by their partner through the conscious or unconscious gaining, regaining or maintaining power through the repetitive overt or subtle acts and messages that control or attempt to control, which negatively affects the abused partner's emotions or self-value in the long term. (Lammers et al. 2005, p. 87).

They maintain that it is important to differentiate emotionally abusive behaviour from emotional abuse. Although there may be transitory feeling of emotional pain due to emotionally abusive behaviour, it is the patterned and recurring experience that makes it abusive with long-term negative consequences (Follingstad and DeHart 2000; Marshall 1994, 1996; Loring 1994). The context of NPA is significant, with abuse that occurs in public viewed as more abusive than when the same behaviour is performed in private (Follingstad 2007).

The vast majority of abuse is non-physical (Dueckman 2012; Outlaw 2009), with NPA by a current partner being four times as common as physical violence (Tjaden and Thoennes 2000). However, prevalence rates can vary due to the disagreement about what constitutes emotional abuse (Mohr and Barner 2012). The recognition of NPA within intimate relationships is recent (Outlaw 2009), and victims often report that forms of NPA have a more devastating effect on them than physical injury (Outlaw 2009; Seff et al. 2008; Ro and Lawrence 2007; Bancroft 2002; Loring 1994). Women can experience NPA for years without recognizing their partner's behaviour as abusive (Carlyle et al. 2008; O'Hagan 2006, 1995; Zink et al. 2003; Miller and Stiver 1997). They can be ashamed (Dueckman 2012; James and MacKinnon 2010), covering up abuse, or may convince themselves that they are not being abused (Dueckman 2012; James and MacKinnon 2010). NPA may act as a warning sign for physical abuse and is common amongst those experiencing PA. The most salient feature of emotional abuse is its insidious nature (Outlaw 2009; Lachkar 2000; Lammers et al. 2005), with many types of emotionally abusive behaviour appearing socially acceptable, for example, abusive remarks disguised as jokes (Lammers et al. 2005). Evans (2000) points out that verbal abuse is built into our culture with: one-upmanship, putting down, countering, criticizing and intimidating accepted as fair games by many. Emotional abuse may not be recognized early on in a relationship, or by others when the abuser adopts the 'charm syndrome', exploiting their charisma to get their way and manipulate victims into compliance (Hoyle 2013; Evans 1993; Horley 1991). This may explain why there is often shock among family and friends when the abuser is 'outed'. The abuser can switch from charm to rage, which can be confusing. Outsiders may think he is wonderful. Consequently, the victim can think that she is imagining the abuse and start to doubt her own judgement (Hoyle 2013; Horley 1991). Women can be conditioned to believe that they are at fault for the treatment they receive, not recognizing that they are a victim (Evans 2000; Sims 2008; Engel 2002; Hirigoyen 1998). Not identifying abuse can negatively affect victims' ability to defend against and recover from the abuse (Marshall 1996). Self-blame often remains well beyond the end of the relationship (Dutton and Painter 1993). NPA can be dismissed as relationship conflict, or overlooked when there is no overt conflict or physical assault. A common sentiment among victims is, wishing that the abuser would hit them so they would have concrete proof of abuse or a perceived justifiable excuse to leave the relationship (Dueckman 2012). NPA is motivated by the need to control (Outlaw 2009). Even when physical violence has stopped for many years, abusers may still use NPA to ensure ongoing submission and compliance (James and MacKinnon 2010; Mezey et al. 2002). Although age is negatively related to rates of physical abuse, it is not to rates of NPA, with men increasingly relying on NPA in later years to maintain power and control rather than physical violence (Mezey et al. 2002).

James and MacKinnon (2010) describe three levels of NPA: verbal, emotional and psychological, with a significant overlap between these three levels. Second degree emotional abuse usually incorporates first degree verbal abuse, and third degree psychological abuse usually incorporates emotional abuse. Miller (2006) has found that jealousy, shouting, swearing and insisting on knowing the victim's whereabouts at all times, were among the most common forms of controlling behaviours. Emotional abuse is now believed to exist independently of PA (Lammers et al. 2005). According to Loring (1994), NPA can be overt (such as openly demeaning and defacing, verbal remarks, put-downs or constant criticisms), or covert forms of abuse which are more subtle and hidden, but are equally as devastating. NPA can involve comments and actions intended to undermine the victim's self-respect and self-worth and may include: complaints, insults/put-downs, name calling, public embarrassment and accusations (Miller and Stiver 1997), rejection, humiliation and degradation, threats and terrorization (Follingstad and DeHart 2000), yelling, screaming, intentionally withdrawing, or withholding emotional support or affection (Tolman 1989), infantilization, and being given the 'silent treatment' (Seff et al. 2008). Behaviours designed to hurt a person's feelings about themselves, i.e. verbal abuse, wounding around sexuality and attractiveness, public humiliation and creating a hostile environment were found to be rated worse than expressions of jealousy or attempts to control decision making (Follingstad 2011).

Psychological abuse undermines the victim's security of their own logic and reasoning. A victim can become economically dependent on the abuser who can then decide if the victim is to receive any monies, and how much. This is often inadequate to meet household expenses (Miller and Stiver 1997). Stark (2007) talks of coercive control in which victims are frequently deprived of: support from family and friends, money, food, access to communication or transportation, and other survival resources. Victims can become isolated (Miller and Stiver 1997). Behaviours can intend to produce compliance or subservience, to isolate from personal and social resources, or to elicit conformity to traditional gender roles (Tolman 1989). Behaviours designed to keep a person in an inferior position, without others to help maintain their self-concept or hurt one's feelings after actions that were sadistic and threatening, were rated the most serious (Follingstad 2011). Intimidating behaviour can be used to enforce women's compliance. It is this overt form of non-physical control that is most closely aligned with physical violence (Lammers et al. 2005). Marshall (1996) calls this 'symbolic violence', and the effect on victims is often that of fear. Women exposed to overt EA, who are aware of their subordinate status and the unacceptability of their partners' behaviour, can view their submission as a means of survival rather than a character trait (Lammers et al. 2005).

The effects of NPA can be the erosion of the self, feelings of despair, confusion, sadness, loneliness (Loring 1994); inferiority and worthlessness (Woods 1999), which undermine a sense of control (Patton and Mannison 1995). Feelings of inadequacy due to emotional isolation, separation or the threat of it may turn to feelings of shame (Mullally 2000). Self-*suicide* confidence can be lost when women are treated in a paternalistic way, as if they are immature or in of need guidance. Women felt lonely when their personal needs weren't considered, and they were not seen as individuals with needs and desires of their own (Lammers et al. 2005). Due to damage to their self-esteem, a victim's beliefs, values and needs may be given up if they clash with the needs or expectations of their partner, with the hope of becoming acceptable to them (Lammers et al. 2005; Engel 2002). Victims may have suicidal thoughts (Loring 1994), feelings of hopelessness or profound sadness (Lammers et al. 2005), often not knowing why, which Hochschild (1983) calls 'the problem with no name' – a type of unidentifiable depression. Subtle abuse can be more effective in controlling a victim than physical violence. Confusion is caused when an abuser displays caring as well as abusive behaviour, with actions not matching their words, such as when a woman's perception of things is constantly denied, or the behaviour is subtly demeaning, and external reasons are not found for feeling bad. When no understandable or predictable cause can be found for the change in her partner's behaviour, then women may believe that they have caused it, and as a consequence, would do anything to please them. The effect of an abuser's constantly changing behaviour is linked to a diminished sense of identity, severely reduced self-esteem, and uncertainty about one's own perceptions. If criticism is at a low level, it is difficult for women to grasp that they are being demeaned, and those who are unaware that they are being abused can doubt their own sanity (Lammers et al. 2005; Marshall 1994). Abusers will deny, minimize, or justify their behaviour, leaving the victim distraught as well as confused (James and MacKinnon 2010). Engel (2002), Hirigoyen (1998), Miller (1995) and Evans (1993) describe brain-washing, or mind control techniques, such as social isolation, provocation of fear, alternating kindness with threats of disequilibrium and the induction of guilt and self-blame. Promoting dependency and identity erosion can be used against women to debilitating effect. Hyper-vigilance is also a common effect for those who experience sudden outbursts for no apparent reason or drastic mood swings and inconsistent responses (Engel 2002).

Older women report significant physical, as well as mental health, consequences when experiencing ongoing abuse (James and MacKinnon 2010; Fisher and Regan 2006; Zink et al. 2003; Loring 1994). Even if women do not recognize that they are experiencing abuse, they may seek treatment for chronic symptoms that they do not realize are a result of the stress and trauma that they experience (Loring 1994). Women can suffer from PTSD with symptoms such as anxiety, nightmares, intrusive thoughts and persistent painful memories (James and MacKinnon 2010; Miller and Stiver 1997). Trauma responses are related not only to the intensity of the events experienced, but also to their duration. Long-standing, or repeated, exposure to traumatic events that involve extended periods of time and a sense of 'prolonged and sickening anticipation', have a significant psychological impact (Terr 1991 p. 10). The traumatic response may be less clearly related to a single event, than to the gradual wearing away of a person's ability to feel comfortable and safe within relationships, and may destroy the desire and capacity for relationships (Sorsoli 2004). Psychologists have come to understand the capacity and desire for relationships is central to human development, and may affect the way trauma is experienced (Miller 1976/1986). Development occurs within, and through, relationships which can foster psychological growth, or be predominantly harmful (Sorsoli 2004). Damage to a person's self-value and self-confidence, due to NPA, may result in a diminished identity (Kirkwood 1993) which is related to a loss of self-esteem (Lammers et al. 2005). An abuser may undermine their partner's sense of self by attacking her personhood, ignoring, demeaning, belittling, ridiculing personal traits or criticizing behaviour (Sackett and Saunders 1999). A strong sense of identity has been found to be more fundamentally related to one's well-being than high self-esteem (Kirkwood 1993). Women who are continually made to feel unworthy of love or fair treatment, may start focusing inwards to try and make sense of their abuser-partner's behaviour, and begin to feel inadequate (Loring 1994; Marshall 1996). They may internalize their abuser's accusations of 'bad', 'mad' or 'inadequate' (James and MacKinnon 2010). Those who do not have a solid sense of self or do not value themselves highly are more susceptible to being controlled (Lammers et al. 2005). Those who are emotionally abused can experience negative psychological outcomes long after the relationship has finished (Reed and Enright 2006). However, there can be positive changes such as personal growth, enhanced relationships and a changed view of the self after adversity, which is named by Linley and Joseph (2004) as adversarial growth.

Evans (1993) believes that the oppression of verbal abuse is so deeply woven into the fabric of society, that it often goes unnoticed. Before the 1970s, abuse was viewed as a private

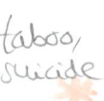

taboo,
suicide

affair, and there is still a perceived lack of social responsibility around the area, with a tolerance of all forms of NPA reflected by the silence surrounding it. This is exemplified by the lack of recognition by journalists, with abuse being presented in many articles as taking only a physical form (Carlyle et al. 2008). It becomes doubly invisible as there are no visible wounds and the media actually frames NPA as physical. The result is that the impact, and the resulting pain, are obscured (Sims 2008), and NPA remains unrecognized by those in an abusive situation (Carlyle et al. 2008). Our culture is patriarchal, viewing women as intrinsically less worthy than men who hold the power (Miller 1976/1986). This affects the way we make sense of the world, our experiences, and the experiences of others (Becker 1998). Social and political structures support gender inequality, with oppressive gender roles and characteristics seen as natural, therefore, unchangeable, and this can obscure the emotional abusiveness of gendered practices. Men are expected to rule and dominate women, who take the role of helpers and care-givers. The law has upheld the patriarchal view of women and their place in the world.

> Under the 1860 Law of Coverture a husband was legally responsible for his wife and children and he could, therefore, physically and verbally chastise them to control their behaviour. The attitude of police to domestic violence was summed up by the Metropolitan Police Commissioner 24 years ago when he linked it with stray dogs describing both as 'rubbish work for police officers'.
>
> Marital rape was only made a criminal act in 1991 (www.womensaid.org.uk/core/core_picker/download. asp?id=1859).

The law is only now beginning to recognize NPA. Following calls from local authorities, police and voluntary organizations, the definition of domestic abuse has been widened to cover psychological intimidation and controlling behaviour. This change was implemented in March 2013 (http://www.bbc.co.uk/news/education-19640257) and recognizes that behavioural patterns such as intimidation, isolation and depriving victims of their financial independence and material possessions, can constitute abuse (Hoyle 2013). Psychological abuse will now be recognized in rape cases, with sentencing taking into account the severity of the psychological effects. Johnson (2005) argues that most discussion of gender-based violence is focused on individuals, but maintains that we should examine aspects of the patriarchal social system. Organizations, such as the Church, with its traditional views of male-dominated roles both within the Church and the marriage relationships, can serve to perpetuate the sense of power-lessness an abused woman feels. Many believe that women should be submissive to their husbands who should be head of the household. Women can feel guilt in leaving a marriage because of the teaching that divorce is a sin, and as a Christian you should forgive (Dueckman 2012). Difficulties with the subject of emotional abuse may also arise from the culturally dominant narratives about emotion, and the denigration of emotional pain as a legitimate form of suffering (Sorsoli 2004). Looking at a wide range of traumatic experiences, including emotional abuse, it is easier to understand trauma in terms of physical events, with claims of trauma only presumed accurate when they were consistent with the understanding that pain and suffering is caused only by physical harm. This supports the idea that 'getting one's feelings hurt' automatically implies weakness (Brown 1995). Women's belief that they have been emotionally hurt by their partner, may be negated, minimized, or rejected, and the expression of this belief may cause them to be negatively labelled (Lammers et al. 2005). Allowable emotional expression differs by gender. Women are expected to express a wider range of emotions, but are deemed 'weak' for being 'emotional', and accused of being immoral or unjust (Gilligan 1996) and even pathologized (Loring and Powell 1988).

Battered women tend to be more able to admit that they have been emotionally abused, as if the physical harm gives them the permission to suffer from emotional harm (Loring 1994). Trauma survivors often say that what they experienced 'could've been worse', and condemn themselves for the depth and intensity of their feelings, or find other reasons, often involving an inherent weakness of self, for their pain. The cultural narrative of having one's feelings hurt is no big deal, and that emotional suffering is a sign of weakness, or immaturity, is a great impediment to survivors, as it can stop empathy. It is when we understand the depth of the human desire for connection and relationship, that abusive relationships can be understood and seem logical (Sorsoli 2004; Miller 1976/1986).

The reasons for staying in an NPA relationship can vary, and can be for financial dependence, not wanting to disturb their children, not wanting to break up the family unit, the reaction that friends, or family, may have, the change being too overwhelming (Dueckman 2012), having no social support, being scared to leave, threats from partner, or having a sense of love and attachment (Sims 2008; Dueckman 2012). Even realizing that their relationship is detrimental to them, women may feel unable to leave due to their self-esteem being seriously eroded, and their feelings of worthlessness and loss of confidence (Lammers et al. 2005). They may be emotionally dependent on the person through a process known as 'traumatic bonding' (Bancroft 2002). Christian women may stay to avoid the admission of marriage failure, and possible rejection by the Church (Dueckman 2012), or believe that marriage is for life (Lammers at al. 2005). Women may see behaviours such as wanting constant attention, not allowing time with friends and family and jealousy as signs of love rather than early warning signs of power and control issues (Power 2004). It is possible that unresolved negative childhood experiences can play a part in a woman's vulnerability to emotional exploitation (Lammers at al. 2005). Defences and coping systems such as dissociation, repression, denial and identification with the aggressor, may be mobilized to deal with the trauma, and may lead to distinct character changes (Terr 1991). Women may disconnect emotionally due to being constantly criticized, discounted or demeaned by their partners, which can result in loneliness (Lammers et al. 2005). The beliefs and attitudes about intimate relationships that women have, can influence their interpretation of their partner's behaviour (DeHart et al. 2010). The first step to leaving an abusive relationship is for a woman to become aware that she has changed over time in ways that she considers to be negative, and then connect this to her partner's behaviour. This may result in a change in energy levels that can manifest as anger or fear. Long-suppressed feelings may erupt and seem to come from nowhere (Kirkwood 1993). Anger is a significant part of recovery. Expressions of anger depend upon how much emotional pain women have experienced and if they feel safe to express it (Lammers et al. 2005). The final step towards personal power comes when women have emotionally disconnected from their partner, described by Loring (1994) as 'disattachment'. Letting go in this way can increase their personal power, and they can become less dependent on their partner's behaviour to feel good (Lammers et al. 2005). When they do leave, they may have no sense of what is important to them, or how they feel about anything. They may have discarded personal morals, ethics and opinions to avoid fights in the relationship, and their sense of self may have been consumed by their controlling partner (Loring 1994).

The literature demonstrates that NPA is so ingrained in the culture that it is often unseen and unrecognized. Victims are often confused, blame themselves for the situation and change themselves in response to the abusive behaviour. The term NPA covers a wide range of behaviour that aims to control the other person in the relationship. There is also a wide range of effects with a loss of confidence and the loss of a sense of self being common. *More loss*
Desire to avoid loss → internal conflict

Participants

Purposive sampling was used to select participants who conformed to the criteria needed for participation. Due to the sensitive nature of the research, criteria were chosen to protect the participants. They had to have access to counselling and supervision in case of unresolved issues. They were not to have experienced NPA for the past two years and had to believe that they had resolved issues raised by their experience so that they had the necessary distance from issues, and could be interviewed without becoming overwhelmed. They also had to be robust enough to be interviewed. Counsellors were chosen because of the level of personal development that they are required to undergo as a necessary part of their training to be Counsellors. Their training may have enabled NPA to be recognized where it had previously been unseen. The sample size was four participants, giving enough data to examine similarities and differences between participants, while at the same time not so big that there a danger of being overwhelmed by the data (Smith et al. 2009). The participants self-selected and received full information about the study before agreeing to be interviewed. There was no pressure to *Ethics* participate, thereby, avoiding ethical issues. Each participant

132

was given a pseudonym to protect their anonymity. Details about the participants are in Table 7.

	Abby	Becky	Cath	Dot
Age	50–60 years	50–60 years	40–50 years	40–50 years
Age difference	5–10 years	Less than 5 years	Less than 5 years	Less than 5 years
How long in rel.	5–10 years	10–20 years	5–10 years	2–5 years
Age when left	Under 30 years	40–50 years	Under 30 years	30–40 years

Table 7. Description of the participants.

Data collection

A selection of counselling agencies was used to advertise for participants. Before the interview, participants signed consent forms agreeing to be interviewed. Interviews were semi-structured, based on the following questions:

- Your age.
- Your level of education and employment at the time the abuse took place.
- The nature of your relationship.
- The nature of the abuse and the effects on you.
- How the abuse was recognized.
- The reasons you gave for the behaviour before it was recognized.
- The reasons you were vulnerable to being abused.
- Any negative or positive coping skills you had.
- Barriers to seeking help.
- Reasons you stayed or left.

The interviews were digitally recorded, and the transcript pertaining to that participant was checked by the participant.

Findings

Four master themes were found comprising eight master themes (see Table 8).

Major theme 1: The Insidious Nature of NPA
    Sub-theme 1.1: Deception:
    Sub-sub-theme 1.1.1: Partner's charm: The behaviour of an abuser can be deceiving as they are often, initially, very 'charming' as described by Abby, Cath and Dot. Charm can be a 'hook' into a relationship as it was with Abby. Charming is often how others experience the abuser: *"… they're a very charismatic person, they're a pleasing, willing, engaging, charismatic person. It's interesting because probably that was a hook, into my situation to hook me in"* (Abby). For Cath, *"he was very charming"*; for Dot, *"everybody loves him … he was a very charismatic man, very charming, very friendly"*. Becky's situation is slightly different, in that the abuse was tied up with alcohol abuse by her husband. Although she did not describe her husband as charming, she expressed it as they were very sociable when they first met. She also describes how his behaviour changed at weekends when he *"behaved like any normal father"*, in contrast to during the week when he drank after work and came home drunk. *"It was just a very sociable relationship … I suppose it was like Hyde in the week and Jekyll at weekends which put me on an emotional see-saw"*.

    Sub-sub-theme 1.1.2: Covered up: Abusive remarks may be covered up under the guise of being a joke, either by the perpetrator or those on the receiving end, as was the case for Abby – *"it's classed as a joke and you seem to be the butt of the joke"*, and Cath, *"… sometimes when he belittled us in front of people, they*

Master themes	Sub-themes	Sub-sub-themes and sub-sub-sub themes
1 - Insidious Nature of NPA	1.1 Deception	1.1.1 Partner's charm 1.1.2 Covered up

	1.2 How NPA is experienced	1.2.1 As a unique experience
		1.2.2 Symbolic violence
		1.2.3 As a common experience
		  1.2.3.1 verbally attacked
		  1.2.3.2 constant vigilance
		  1.2.3.3 feeling ill
		  1.2.3.4 isolation
		  1.2.3.5 confusion

2 - The Impact of NPA on the self	2.1 Self-identity	2.1.1 Control 2.1.2 Loss of self 2.1.3 Blaming self
	2.2 Changes in self image	2.2.1 Lasting damage 2.2.2 Gains
3 - The Traps of NPA	3.1 Perpetuating NPA	3.1.1 Cultural norms 3.1.2 Dependency within the relationship
	3.2 The individual's vulnerability to NPA	3.2.1 Individual's underlying vulnerability 3.2.2 Role of the mother 3.2.3 Coping strategies
4 - The Awareness of NPA	4.1 Reflection	4.1.1 Hindsight 4.1.2 Comparing
	4.2 Awareness	4.2.1 Participant's own awareness 4.2.2 Other's awareness of the relationship

Table 8. Master themes with the sub-themes, sub-sub-themes and sub-sub-sub-themes.

would look at us and I would laugh it off and go 'he's just joking man, he doesn't mean it'" Abby covered up her feelings due to the abusive remarks: *"... you have to create another face or another persona that you're OK when deep down, it hurts".* For Dot, this was the same, *"I just kept up appearances for the first four years".* Dot also gave alternative reasons for the behaviour, helping to keep it unseen: *"I started using the excuses he used for his behaviour".* Cath compromised her own integrity and personal standards which she found *"horrific"*, having to back up her ex-husband's lies as this was expected of her and there would be consequences if she did not: *"He would sit in circles of friends and say things that were totally untrue and ask me to back him up … I detest lying, but I couldn't see a way out of it".*

Sub-theme 1.2: How NPA is experienced:

Sub-sub-theme 1.2.1: As a unique experience: There was a wide range of abusive behaviour carried out on the participants, and the scale of this varied. Verbal abuse was common. Abby described these as *"little comments … innuendos".* Cath stated that, *"he belittled me constantly".* Cath had unrealistic expectations demanded of her: *"I was the wage earner, bottle washer, everything else you could think of … while he sat at home and did nothing".* Dot also experienced a range of abusive behaviour, including having accusations made against her when she was late home from work: *"… was an accusation I was actually having an affair with someone from work and he even made me show him the tooth in my mouth that had been filled".* Becky's ex-husband's behaviour was linked to alcohol and being drunk. He was not available to her emotionally or psychologically after drinking, and she was left at home alone as he stayed out: *"there was no conversation, we didn't have any adult conversation … waiting for him or waiting for an adult to come home, but he didn't come home".* The abuse escalated for the participants. Abby stated, *"… little quirk comments and then moving on and them becoming more derogatory and more challenging".* For Cath: *"it escalated into sexual abuse",* and for Dot, *"the abuse escalated while I was pregnant".* Abuse escalated

Not present (not alive)

at different times of the year for Becky due to her husband's drinking: *"it was worse leading up to Christmas"*. There was a wish from Abby who had experienced verbal abuse, that the abuse *"would get worse"*, because *"when it's little it doesn't seem worth bothering about"*. Whether the abusive behaviour occurred in public, private, or both, differed for the participants. For Abby, it was *"predominantly around when my ex-partner could have an audience"*, and for Cath, it was *"public and private"*. The occurrence of the abusive behaviour also varied. Cath stated that, *"every single day he put me down"*. For Dot, the abusive *"episodes"* were" *quite far apart and in between he was back to who he was when I met him"*.

Sub-sub-theme 1.2.2: Symbolic violence: Cath and Dot experienced symbolic violence with the implicit threat that the violence could be turned towards them. As a result, they were afraid, and experienced the most extreme effects in comparison to Abby and Becky. Cath stated that, *"he would throw things, he pulled a door off its hinges and things like that … I was thinking of taking my life. I was always frightened that it would turn to me"*. Dot stated that, *"I'd be pinned to a wall with him shouting in my face"* and replied *"Yes"* when asked if she was afraid in the relationship. *"I can't even try and explain to someone the mental turmoil and the all time low that I was at"*.

Sub-sub-theme 1.2.3: As a common experience:

Sub-sub-sub-theme 1.2.3.1: verbally attacked: Although the participants did not all have the same abusive behaviour acted against them, all experienced verbal abuse, with this taking various forms. Abby was *"ridiculed, humiliated, put down as and when"*. Becky and Cath experienced criticism and were undermined. Becky stated, *"he would belittle me about the things that I chose and my decision-making"*, and Cath stated, *"I was never good enough, and everything I did was wrong"*. Dot experienced abusive anger and name calling: *"calling me names, quite nasty sexual names, shouting them in my face"*.

Sub-sub-sub-theme 1.2.3.2: constant vigilance: Abuse is often unpredictable and unexpected and resulted in constant vigilance for all of the participants. For Abby it was, *"You don't know when it's going to happen"*, and for Becky, it was a *"constant watching him, constant vigilance"*. Cath described it as *"walking on egg shells constantly"*, and Dot stated that, *"he would come in and he was like thunder and I would really have to monitor that"*.

Sub-sub-sub-theme 1.2.3.3: feeling ill: Constant vigilance can result in stress with the accompanying physical symptoms. Physical symptoms can be reported but not connected to the experience of abuse as it is often unrecognized by those who experience it. Abby, Cath and Dot all reported physical and mental symptoms of stress.

Sub-sub-sub-theme 1.2.3.4: isolation: Isolation was a common experience with all participants. Becky, Cath and Dot were isolated due to not having contact with others. For Becky and Dot, this was enforced on them, whereas for Cath *"felt very isolated, very much on my own"*. It was due to Cath being in a foreign country, but that is not to say it would not have been enforced if deemed necessary. Becky stated, *"I was on my own with a small baby just feeling really lonely nobody to go to"*. Dot described it as, *"becoming isolated from them, and it wasn't until a lot later when I began reflecting on things that I realised he'd instigated a lot of that"*. Abby experienced isolation, not because she did not have people around her, but because they didn't understand her experience: *"… it can be very isolating sometimes because who can you go to, who can you turn to, how do you explain?"*

Sub-sub-sub-theme 1.2.3.5: confusion: Confusion was common with all participants and was created in various ways. Abby had her reactions to the verbal abuse discounted and ascribed to a characteristic of her personality. As her experience was not validated, she became so confused that she wished she could have had tangible proof of the reality of what was happening. Abby stated, *"you're being over sensitive, it wasn't meant like that'… questioning yourself, are you going mad. It would've been good to have taped and analysed it"*. The invalidation of one's experience, explaining away of behaviour; countering what is said and denial of the behaviour is so confusing that Cath would agree to her ex-husband's interpretation of reality. *"He would twist it and turn it and in the end I was like, yes you're right it's my fault"*. Dot expressed the confusion she felt as, *"there's something about unpredictability and inconsistency that completely messes with your head"*. Becky expressed her confusion as reading a lot to make sense of what was happening in her relationship.

Major theme 2: The Impact of NPA on the Self
Sub-theme 2.1: Self identity:
Sub-sub-theme 2.1.1: Control: The commonality with all of the abusive behaviour was that it was used for the purpose of control, as expressed by Cath: *"… he controlled me and my choice was taken away and that was one of the biggest things"*. Control was expressed in different ways by the participants. Abby expressed it as the way she was treated: *"I was treated like a child, a protected child"*. Cath tried, unsuccessfully, to stand up to her ex-husband: *"I tried to say 'No', it didn't matter. He was in charge"*. Controlling behaviour may not be noticed in the beginning of the relationship, but this was not the case for Dot: *"he dictated the pace of the relationship not me"*. Although there was no overt control of Becky by her husband, his drinking impacted on her being able to go out and see friends as he needed to look after their children. *"I'd have to make a judgement as to whether I could leave the children with him or not"*.

139

Sub-sub-theme 2.1.2: Loss of self: Loss of self is a significant effect of being abused, with Abby, Cath and Dot expressing this. Cath expressed the speed at which this happened while for Dot it was a maladaptive coping mechanism. Abby stated that, *"the death of your identity was strongly connected to that person".* Cath said, *"I can't believe how quickly I lost my identity".* Dot stated, *"I lost touch with who I was and tried to start becoming who he wanted me to be".*

Sub-sub-theme 2.1.3: Blaming self: All of the participants had a distorted perception of the reasons for the abuse. This can be due to having their experience being invalidated and the confusion this causes. Consequently they looked to themselves for the cause, internalizing the blame that was attributed to them by their ex-partners. Dot said, *"I started believing it was me as well and trying to change myself ... he'd call me things like, 'You're mad, you're mad', and I used to think, well maybe I am because of that".* This was not the case for Becky as she believed she was to blame due to a belief she had about herself: *"didn't deserve someone to come home to me".*

Sub-theme 2.2: Changes in self image:

Sub-sub-theme 2.2.1: Lasting damage: Three of the participants believed that there was lasting damage due to the abusive relationship which they had all left many years ago. As Dot became aware of issues due to the past, she was able to work through them with the hope that with time any damage would be dealt with.

Sub-sub-theme 2.2.2: Gains: There were gains after leaving the relationship for three of the participants. Dot named this as *"post-traumatic growth",* and linked the experience to her present happiness: *"I think if I hadn't of had that experience, I don't know if I'd be as happy as this now ... helped me realise who I am".* Becky came to the realization that she no longer needed a man in her life, *"I'm OK on my own",* whereas before the relationship this was a driving force in her forming relationships. Increased confidence was a common gain by participants with Abby stating *"you become a stronger person"*. Cath's experience was different, it was not so much that she gained from the experience but that she was able to be herself again: *"I'm back to who I would've been and I'm comfortable in my skin again"*.

Master theme 3: The Traps of NPA
Sub-theme 3.1: Perpetuating NPA:
Sub-sub-theme 3.1.1: Cultural norms: NPA is ingrained in the culture as found by Abby: *"it's in the media and it's pervasive throughout everywhere"*. Becky found that the sanctity of her marriage vows, and what it meant to be a Christian, could have stopped her leaving her marriage: *"He said what kind of a Christian was I just to break my marriage vows like that, now that could've got to me"*. Cath learnt what to expect from a relationship from her parents: *"I thought this was what a relationship was"*, while Dot learnt the cultural norms *"from my parents' relationship, you stick at a marriage and you try and make it work regardless"*.

Sub-sub-theme 3.1.2: Dependency within the relationship: Participants could be dependent on their partners emotionally, financially or socially. It was not only the participants who expressed being dependent, for Dot it was her ex-husband's expression of dependency that manipulated her into staying when she went to leave: *"I'd go to leave and he'd change his demeanour immediately and become like a crying baby almost begging me, being exactly who he was when I met him"*.

Sub-theme 3.2: The individual's vulnerability to NPA:
Sub-sub-theme 3.2.1: Individual's underlying vulnerability: The participants were vulnerable to an abusive relationship and this was expressed in a variety of ways. Becky and Dot did not have a strong sense of self when they met their

ex-husbands. Becky stated, *"I came from a position of being lacking ... I think I was vulnerable to relationships which weren't the best because it was like any relationship was better than none"*. Dot said, *"I didn't have a very strong sense of self"*. Dot had *"unresolved issues"* due to a violent attack that happened before she met her ex-husband which were exploited and used against her. Abby had a belief of what it was to be a wife and mother, *"putting your needs before everybody else can feel a bit selfish"*. Cath fell in love in a foreign country and saw things *"through rose tinted glasses"*. When she married *"it was like a fairy tale marriage"*.

Sub-sub-theme 3.2.2: Role of the mother: Becoming a mother was significant for all of the participants for a variety of reasons. For Abby, the dynamics of her relationship changed: *"There was a shift in the relationship because I was a mother"*. Being a mother gave Becky more resilience and was a reason to stay in the relationship: *"if it's for the children then I can put up with more ... my children wouldn't grow up with their Mother and Father together and I didn't want that"*. Cath changed the focus of her attention which may have been a coping mechanism as the abuse was pushed to the background. Her children were also the reason she left the relationship: *"I focused on them ... I would've still been in that relationship had I not had children I know that for a fact"*. Dot *"became an overnight mother"* when she became a step-mother, and it was this that stopped her leaving the relationship. However, becoming pregnant was the start of self-care as she worried for herself and the baby: *"I started going to yoga and tried my best to take care of myself"*. When asked what gave her the push to leave, Dot replied, *"my own daughter"*.

Sub-sub-theme: Coping strategies: All of the participants developed various coping strategies. They ranged from Becky diverting attention to the children: *"I just focused on the children"*, to Cath shutting down emotionally and blocking things out: *"I really withdrew, I was a shell, I had no emotion"* and

142

"try and block everything out"; or from Becky gaining strength via a belief *"belief in God gave me extra strength"*, to Abby protecting herself through distancing *"develop another screen to your persona"* and Dot changed becoming what was expected of her as she *"tried to start becoming who he wanted me to be"*.

Master theme 4: The Awareness of NPA
Sub-theme 4.1: Reflection:
Sub-sub-theme 4.1.1: Hindsight: Time was a significant feature for the participants in recognizing that they had experienced abusive behaviour, with none of the participants recognizing it initially until, as Dot describes, *"I started seeing things differently"*. Recognition can be a gradual process as it was for Dot: *"It wasn't an overnight process"*. It can be a shock when the abuse is recognized. Cath stated, *"I just didn't see it. I look back now and I think my God what was I doing"*. The situation for Becky was slightly different. She was always aware that her husband drank, but she was not aware that she experienced abusive behaviour until she saw a poster and reflected back. Becky said, *"that was me but I never till that day connected it with abuse"*. It was also via information that Dot began to recognize the abuse: *"I picked up a leaflet and it was from Women's Aid and it had a check list on the back of it"*. Time is significant as abusive behaviour can escalate, so becoming more recognizable. It was changes in Abby's behaviour that started her recognition, *"to a point when it does your bloody head in. Your brain can only take so much"*.

Sub-sub-theme 4.1.2: Comparing: The use of comparison, aids the recognition of abuse. For participants, it happened in a variety of ways. Abby compared others' relationships with her own *"different to what's happening in mine"*; seeing fear in Cath's children alerted her: *"I saw it reflected in them"*. Becky compared her own experience with and without the presence of her ex-husband *"he was in prison for that two months ... I felt a lot lighter"* and Dot compared how her behaviour had changed: *"Suddenly became this Muslim woman who wasn't allowed to speak to anybody"*.

Sub-theme 4.2: Awareness:

Sub-sub-theme 4.2.1: Participant's own awareness: Due to their experience of NPA, participants developed an awareness of the signs of an abusive relationship when previously they may not have identified it. Abby was *"very aware of it and it's funny you can see it in others"*. Cath stated, *"I'm more in tune now with how people can be in that type of situation"*. Dot developed an awareness of the characteristics of abusive men: *"you could almost be talking about the same man"*, while Becky looked at her future: *"I could see my life from that point not changing"*.

Sub-sub-theme 4.2.2: Other's awareness of the relationship: Other's awareness of the abusive relationship could be completely distorted due to the insidious nature of abuse. Abby's friends thought, *"you had the power"*. The abuser may have covered up their behaviour in public. Cath stated that, *"everybody thought that the relationship was great and he was fantastic"*. Dot said, *"they all thought he was very nice"*. Becky explored the reasons for her husband's behaviour with friends putting it down to his drinking: *"with friends I would explore the possible reasons together"*. Abby found her situation difficult to explain to friends: *"it's a difficult thing to explain because it's so subtle"*. As abusive behaviour can appear sociably acceptable, Abby's friends thought the problem lay with characteristics of her personality for which she needed medication: *"what you're on about 'cause that's the norm for me, I don't believe it or it wasn't meant, it wasn't intentional. It kind of perpetuates this notion that a bit over the ordinary ... you're a bit anxious and you need to get some medication for it"*.

Discussion

I will structure the discussion under the headings of the four master themes:

The insidious nature of NPA: All of the participants were on the receiving end of patterned and recurring NPA which Marshall (1994, 1996) and Loring (1994) say differentiates emotionally abusive behaviour from emotional abuse. The most salient feature of NPA is its insidious nature (Outlaw 2009; Lachkar 2000; Lammers et al. 2005). One of the deceptive behaviours of men who later turn out to be abusive is that they are charming on initial meeting. This quality was reported by three of the participants, with the fourth describing her ex-husband as very sociable. Charisma was described as the hook into the relationship by Abby. The participants' experience is supported by the research, with the behaviour named 'the charm syndrome' and used by perpetrators to get their way, manipulating victims into compliance (Hoyle 2013; Evans 1993; Horley 1991). Participants helped keep the abusive behaviour hidden in public in various ways, as found by Dueckman (2012), James and MacKinnon (2010); Dot gave alternative reasons, justifying and rationalizing her ex-husband's behaviour as well as keeping up appearances. Cath covered up her ex-husband's hurtful remarks, describing them as jokes, and his lies by agreeing with him. Loring (1994) describes how personal morals, ethics and opinions are discarded to avoid fights, as was the case with Cath, and which she found *"horrific"*. Abby covered up her feelings, creating another persona. Abby, being the *"butt of the joke"*, was accepted by others as *"normal"*, confirming Lammers et al.'s (2005) view that many types of emotionally abusive behaviour appears socially acceptable. NPA covers a wide range of behaviour as found by many researchers (e.g. Follingstad 2011; James and MacKinnon 2010; Outlaw 2009; Millar 2006, 1995; Follingstad and DeHart 2000; Lammers et al. 2005; Loring 1994). This was certainly true for the participants, with Abby experiencing comments and innuendos that undermined her; Becky had a husband who was unavailable emotionally or psychologically to her and felt isolated as he did not come home; Cath was belittled, criticized, controlled, had abusive expectations demanded of her and was sexually abused; while Dot was abused verbally, accused of affairs, kept short of money, intimidated and isolated. The participants had very different behaviour acted out towards them, and this agrees with research by Outlaw (2009), that the presence of one form of emotional abuse does not mean that all are present. However, all participants were verbally attacked and criticized, which seems to be in line with James and MacKinnon (2010), that there are three levels of NPA, the first level being verbal abuse. The abuse for three of the participants escalated over time. The abuse escalated for Becky at Christmas as the abuse was linked to her ex-husband's drinking. This aspect of NPA does not seem to have been researched. Research finds that it is common for victims to wish they would be hit so that they would have concrete proof of abuse or a reason to leave the relationship (Dueckman 2012). This is similar to Abby's wish that the abuse would get worse, but her reason was that it didn't seem worth bothering about when it was small. In contrast to the research (Lammers et al. 2005; Marshall 1994) she does realize that the behaviour is 'not right'. NPA can happen in public, in private, or both. Abby found that when the abuse happened in public it was worse than when it happened in private. She was the 'entertainment', felt embarrassed, and did not feel able to challenge the unpleasant remarks; whereas she could in private. Miller (1995) acknowledges that public embarrassment is abusive as it can undermine the victim's self-respect and self-worth, and may explain why, for Abby, it was the context in which the abuse took place that brought about difficulties. This also confirms research by Follingstad (2007) that abuse performed in public is more abusive than when in private. Research describes how abuse can be verbal, but does not describe how it can be for the entertainment of others (Loring 1994). Abuse varied in its regularity for participants: for Cath it was every day; for Dot episodes were quite far apart, escalating when she was pregnant. The research looked at has not addressed the effect of pregnancy on NPA. Two of the participants experienced 'symbolic violence' with the implicit threat to them. This resulted in fear as found by Marshall (1996). They also experienced the most extreme effects due to the abuse, with Cath becoming suicidal, and Dot becoming *"completely messed up"*. The aftermath of the experience also lasted the longest for Cath who still feels *"bitter"* and Dot who feels there *"is still some damage"*. The participants' experience supports Follingstad's (2011) rating of behaviours that were sadistic and threatening, as being the most serious in regard to the effects that they had. Both of the participants were compliant, trying to change themselves to appease their partners, and behave in ways that was expected of them, so supporting the findings of Lammers et al. (2005) who describe how intimidating behaviour can be used in this way, and that it is this type of control that is most closely aligned with physical violence. All participants lost their confidence due to their experience of NPA, an effect that was found to be common in those who experience NPA (Lammers et al. 2005). Three of the participants described being unwell, talked of feeling tired, stressed, unable to concentrate, whilst at the same time not recognizing that this could be due to abuse. This supports research that women report physical and mental health consequences due to abuse (James and MacKinnon 2010; Fisher and Regan 2006; Zink et al. 2003). Stress may be created due to constant vigilance. This was reported by all of the participants, supporting Loring (1994), in that women may seek treatment for chronic symptoms, not realizing that they are the result of stress and trauma. All of the participants found that they had to monitor their partner's behaviour, with Becky and Cath both describing it as *"walking on eggshells"* despite there being very different levels of abuse. This is consistent with research by Engel (2002). It was not until Dot went to the doctor and picked up a leaflet, that she began to recognize that she might be being abused. Cath was the only participant who expressed being suicidal, an effect found by Loring (1994). Cath and Dot experienced the worst abusive behaviour, and the most extreme effects, compared to the other participants, agreeing with Terr's (1991) research that trauma responses are related to the intensity of events experienced, and their duration. Also, Cath was in her relationship for longer than Dot who did not express being suicidal. They both went on to form happy marriages; this differs from research by Sorsoli (2004) who says that the trauma may destroy the capacity and desire for relationships. All of the participants felt lonely. Outlaw (2009) names social abuse as one of four types of abuse in which the person is isolated from their friends, as was the case for three of the participants. Abby's feeling of loneliness was of a different quality, and was to do with her experience of not being understood by others, and so does not fall into the category of social abuse. However, as she was unable to explain her experience, she received no support, did not have her experiences validated by others, and consequently felt lonely (Lammers et al. 2005). All of the participants felt confused for multiple reasons. Three of the participants' ex-partners displayed caring as well as abusive behaviour and three of the women's perceptions were constantly denied – reasons found by Lammers et al. (2005) and Marshall (1994) to be linked to confusion. Confusion was also caused for Abby as her ex-husband denied the abuse, and explained her reactions as being due to a characteristic of her personality. She looked for the reasons within herself, and questioned if she was going mad, as did Dot. This supports James and MacKinnon (2010) who found that this could happen when abusers' accusations of 'mad', 'bad', or 'inadequate', are internalized. All participants felt controlled by their partners, which Outlaw (2009) says may be the motivation behind NPA. For two of the participants there was no overt control. Becky was controlled via her husband's drinking, as he was unreliable and unavailable emotionally and psychologically when drinking. Drinking has not been seen as a controlling behaviour in the research.

The Impact of NPA on the Self: Three of the participants lost a sense of self and this has been found in the research (Kirkwood 1993; Loring 1994; Sackett and Saunders 1999). For Cath this was very quickly, which was not emphasized in the research. Dot changed her behaviour to please her ex-husband, a maladaptive coping mechanism. Lammers et al. (2005) suggest that this is due to the confusion that is caused by abusive behaviour, with women believing it is their fault, and so do anything to please their partner, which in Dot's case, was becoming what he wanted her to be, thus losing touch with who she was. Lammers et al. (2005) also says this can be seen as a means of survival. All of the participants felt they were to blame. This was echoed in the literature (e.g. Evans 2000; Sims 2008; Lammers et al. 2005; Engel 2002; Hirigoyen 1998; Marshall 1994; Dutton and Painter 1993). Abusers can deny, minimize, or justify, their behaviour, leaving victims confused (James and MacKinnon 2010), and those on the receiving end can consequently have a distorted perception of what has happened. If their experience had been negated, victims may internalize, and take responsibility for what has happened. What Miller (1995) writes correlates with Cath and Dot's experiencing. Three of the participants felt damaged by their experience, as supported by Reed and Enright (2006). Sorsoli (2004) points out that development occurs within, and through, relationships, and can be harmful or can foster psychological growth. All of the participants felt that as well as being damaged by the experience of NPA, they also had positive changes, although for Cath it was more a case of finding herself again. Dot put her present happiness down to her experience, which is consistent with research by Linley and Joseph (2004) who call this adversarial growth.

The Traps of NPA: Abby found her abuse to be highly covert and to be pervasive everywhere, and this is supported by the research of Evans (1993) who found that NPA is ingrained in the culture. The Church teaches what is to be expected of marriage and the sanctity of the marriage vows. Women can feel guilty leaving a marriage due to the teaching that this is a sin, and as a Christian you should forgive Dueckman (2012). This was the case with Becky who says that the accusation by her husband, when he was asked to leave, that she was not a good Christian could have got to her. Dot and Cath both had expectations of marriage which they had learnt from their parents which, according to DeHart et al. (2010) could have influenced how they interpreted their partner's behaviour. Research points out that we live in a patriarchal society which influences how we make sense of the world (Becker 1998). Men are expected to dominate women and all of the participants reported being controlled. The law then upholds this view. Although both Cath and Dot's ex-husbands were from overseas, they were both from cultures where patriarchy was evident. Culturally dominant narratives about emotion, and the denigration of emotional pain as a legitimate form of suffering (Sorsoli 2004), are evident when Abby describes how others thought her anxious, a bit over the top, and in need of medication, so being pathologized (Loring and Powell 1998). This supports research by Lammers et al. (2005), that when women express a belief that they have been emotionally hurt, and this is negated, minimized, or rejected, they can be negatively labelled. Dependency was an issue for all participants and took various forms. Three of the participants were dependent on their ex-husbands for different reasons. Abby was dependent emotionally, Becky financially, and Cath as she was in a strange country away from the support of her family. Dot experienced enforced isolation by her ex-husband, as did Cath due to her situation. Although isolation was not forced on Becky, in the sense that she was not allowed out, she was isolated due to her ex-husband's drinking as he was unable to look after their children when he came home drunk. She was also dependent on him financially, staying at home to look after the children. Research does not highlight reasons for isolation but Stark (2007) talks of coercive control when victims are deprived of support of family and friends, as in the case with Becky, Cath and Dot, along with money and food in Cath's case. Abby was emotionally dependent on her ex-husband saying they had a co-dependent relationship. Dot describes how her ex-husband displayed behaviour, such as 'crying', that indicated his dependency and used it to manipulate her into staying in the relationship. This aspect of how the abuser can behave in ways that manipulate the other to stay in the relationship has not come up in the research. Dot was also vulnerable to an abusive relationship due to unresolved issues from her experience of a violent attack, and although she was not a child, research shows that unresolved negative childhood experiences can play a part in a woman's vulnerability to emotional exploitation (Lammers et al. 2005). Two of the participants were vulnerable to becoming involved in an abusive controlling relationship, as they did not have a strong sense of self consistent with research (Lammers et al. 2005). Abby was vulnerable because she felt it was selfish putting her own needs first, a view that would be consistent with the gender roles assigned in a patriarchal society. Cath was vulnerable as she fell in love and went on to have what she thought would be a *"fairy tale marriage"*. She was integrated into her ex-husband's family, as she was abroad, and only saw him occasionally as he worked away. Although she does not explicitly say, she may have experienced behaviours, such as wanting constant attention, not allowing time with friends and family and jealousy as signs of love rather than early warning signs of power and control issues (Power 2004). As she says she saw things through *"rose tinted glasses"*, which may have distorted her view of things. Becoming a mother was significant to all the participants. Abby felt a shift in the relationship when she became a mother. This has not been researched. Children were a reason for Becky and Dot; in Dot's case, her step-daughter, to stay in their relationship which is supported by research (Dueckman 2012); but not for leaving the relationship as Cath did when she had her own child rather than being a mother to her step-daughter. Becky found she could endure more because of her children and this has not been found in the research. Various coping strategies were used by the participants. Abby used a screen to her persona while Becky focused on her children, Cath shut down, and Dot changed herself. Research supports the finding that coping mechanisms of dissociation, repression and disconnecting emotionally are examples of coping strategies that are used and which can lead to character changes (Terr 1991; Lammers et al. 2005).

The Awareness of NPA: Time was a significant feature in the recognition by participants that they were in abusive relationships, and this is supported by research (e.g. Carlyle et al. 2008; O'Hagan 2006, 1995; Zink et al. 2003; Miller 1995). For Abby it was at a point when her head was *"done in"*; for Becky it was many years after the end of the relationship on seeing a poster. Dot only saw the abuse on seeing information from Women's Aid at her GP's practice and she says it took her many years and a lot of help to understand it, and to this day issues can still surface that are connected to the abusive experience. This is consistent with research that says not recognizing abuse may negatively affect a victim's ability to recover (Marshall 1996). Dot's initial reason for going to the GP was that she was pregnant and felt awful, and realized that she needed to start caring for herself. So, inadvertently becoming pregnant was the first step towards caring for herself and recognizing the abuse. Comparison may also help abuse to become recognized. Abby compared her relationship to those of others; Becky compared how she felt when her husband was at home to when he was in prison. Cath recognized the abuse when she saw that her children were frightened of their father and compared it to how she felt, while Dot compared how she was in the present to how she was after becoming what her ex-husband expected, although she does not say that this was the start of the process to leave. Research by Kirkwood (1993) says that the first step to leaving the relationship is when a woman becomes aware of negative changes she has gone through, and connects this to their partner's behaviour as is the case with the participants. Abby and Cath now believe that they would be able to spot an abusive relationship, while Dot recognizes the characteristics of an abusive man. Becky's awareness of her situation changed as she always thought things could improve until the awareness came that they never would. There has been little research to do with victim's awareness in connection with NPA. Outsiders can think the abuser is wonderful as was the case with those who knew Abby, Cath and Dot. This can be confusing as a victim may doubt their own judgement, as was the case with the participants who initially blamed themselves. There can also be shock when the abuser is outed (Hoyle 2013; Evans 1993; Horley 1991). This was not the case for Abby who found that it was so difficult to explain the abuse she experienced because it was so subtle that others did not believe it. Others described the behaviour as normal - dismissing or minimizing it. This confirms the view of NPA as insidious and seemingly socially acceptable (Outlaw 2009; Lachkar 2000; Lammers et al. 2005).

Conclusion

Due to the nature of qualitative research, the sample size is small. Therefore, the results cannot be generalized, although, it can be argued that if an experience is possible, then it is subject to universalization. Language can be considered a limitation, as IPA assumes that the participants' language can capture their experience; however, it can be argued that language constructs, rather than describes, reality, with the same event being able to be described in different ways. IPA can be criticized for not paying enough attention to this constitutive role (Willig 2008). Although it is recognized that men also experience NPA, the sample researched has been kept to women as the cultural and societal expectations for men differ. This is a small-scale study and to include men or same sex partnerships is beyond its scope. However, gender warrants further study, as NPA does not show striking sex differences (Outlaw 2009). The effects, if any, of income, age, cultural background and upbringing, education level, socio-economic status, religious beliefs or childhood experience, age differences between partners and socialized beliefs have not been investigated due to the scale of the research. Although women were volunteering for research, not counselling, their willingness to talk about their 'bad' or 'stressful' relationships implies they may be similar to others who seek relationship counselling. Also, by interviewing only Counsellors, a large section of the population has been excluded from the study and there could be differences in the experience of those who are not Counsellors or those who would not be willing to take part in research.

However, NPA covers a wide range of behaviour which is often hidden, deceptive and manipulative, and clients can come to counselling with issues that may be due to abuse, such as depression and anxiety, but have no understanding that they are being abused. It is important that Counsellors have awareness and understanding of the nature of NPA and the effect it can have on those who experience it. As women who are abused often feel confused, not seeing the behaviour of their spouses as abusive, Counsellors can help to increase their client's understanding of instances of abusive behaviour in their relationship, and of the effect that this has on them. Clients' coping strategies to deal with the abuse, may be explored with attention paid to helping build up the client's confidence, self-esteem and sense of their own identity, which are often destroyed in abusive relationships. Two of the participants became aware that they were being abused after coming across information; this suggests that it would be helpful to have a readily available selection of information describing abusive behaviours in counselling agencies. It would also be helpful for this type of literature to be available in GP's surgeries, as women may attend their GP with physical symptoms which may be a result of NPA.

CHAPTER FIVE

THE IMPACT OF A TRAUMATIC BIRTH ON MOTHERS

Ann Todd

Introduction

Childbirth is a rite of passage, described by many women as a natural, exhilarating and life-enhancing process. Tragically, research suggests that as many as one in three women would describe their birth experience as traumatic and, as a consequence, have experienced post-traumatic stress symptoms (Creedy et al. 2000; Soet et al. 2003; Ayers et al. 2009). Despite these substantial figures, recognition and support for a woman's distress is often unforthcoming. After all, this event has resulted in the birth of a healthy baby, which is something to be celebrated. As a result, recognition of the woman's trauma is often overlooked by medical staff as they commend a good outcome, and perhaps by family and friends as they revel in the excitement of a new baby. There has been an increased interest in birth trauma in the last fifteen years. However, Elmir et al. (2010) point out that there is neither a consistent definition of traumatic birth, nor any systematic way to assess birth trauma. Beck (2004a) would define it as 'actual or threatened serious injury or death to the mother or her infant. The birthing-woman experiences intense fear, helplessness, loss of control and horror' (p. 28). Reid (2011) defines traumatic delivery simply as the woman feeling traumatized by her experience, and is fearful of a subsequent birth. Meanwhile, in the trauma field there has been growing acceptance that what constitutes trauma is subjective (Miliora 1998). Beck's (2004a) study on birth trauma attests to this. Her study found that the participants' perception of their traumatic experience was often viewed as routine by the medical staff. As a result, she concluded that birth trauma 'lies in the eyes of the beholder' (Beck 2004a, p. 28).

Research has reported that in relation to birth trauma, women feel violated, helpless and experience intense fear of death or injury, to either themselves or their baby (Ryding et al. 1998). The negative repercussions can be both ongoing physical and psychological difficulties. Women may experience a myriad of emotions including anger, anxiety, depression and disappointment, and may have an altered sense of self which may leave them feeling inadequate and not whole (Allen 1998; Ayers et al. 2006; Beck 2004a). Research has also informed us that the impact of traumatic birth can affect a woman's attachment to her baby (Ballard et al. 1995; Allen 1998; Soet et al. 2003); affect her relationship with her partner (Fones 1996); and affect decisions about future children (Bailham and Joseph 2003; Beck and Watson 2010). One can see a complex range of emotions and outcomes which affect the woman, and which can ripple into society at large. Indicated rates of Post-Traumatic Stress Disorder (PTSD) in women following a traumatic birth, range from 1.7% (Wijma et al. 1997), to 5.6% (Creedy et al. 2000; Adewuya et al. 2006). However, many more women experience a range of post-traumatic stress symptoms which fall short of a full PTSD diagnosis, the prevalence of which has been measured at up to 33% (Creedy et al. 2000). In mentioning diagnostics, I do not want to pathologize what most now see as a normal reaction to an abnormal event (Carll 2007; Ayers 2004). Nor would I want to confine a woman's experience to a list of symptoms. Post-traumatic stress exists along a continuum, and women's reactions to traumatic birth will be individual rather than standard (White et al. 2006). Whilst most hospitals offer some form of post-natal service, what is offered differs from hospital to hospital. But as post-traumatic stress symptoms do not necessarily appear immediately after the trauma, in fact symptoms may not appear until months later, the mother might well have moved out of the post-natal care system (Peeler et al. 2013). One can imagine how a woman, coming to terms with the demands of a new baby, may be hesitant to seek help. After all, feelings of failure, inadequacy and post-traumatic stress symptoms are at odds with society's expectations of contented motherhood. A mother may be left to process her experience alone.

My interest in this area is a consequence of my own experience of a traumatic birth. After the birth of my daughter, I suffered from HELLP syndrome – a life- threatening complication of pregnancy. Whilst the medical care given to save my life was admirable, my emotional health was given no attention. It may be that little has changed in the intervening years. A recent report by Peeler et al. (2013), suggests that post-natal support is still focused on physical rather than psychological needs. My own experience of birth trauma produced the dichotomous feelings of love and delight in having a daughter; feeling so lucky to be alive; whilst simultaneously feeling inadequate in my failure to have a 'normal' birth; feelings of guilt for the agonizing worry I had put my husband and family through; and an almost unbearable thought that I could have left my child motherless. My experience has given me some awareness of the complexity of emotions, and the difficulty of expressing these at a time that should arguably be the happiest of your life.

My aim in this research is to gain a rich in-depth understanding of the complex meaning of the impact of traumatic childbirth. I sought answers to the following two questions:

- How did my participants process and make sense of their experience?
- How did their lived-experience impact on their lives in the months and years following their birth trauma?

The Birth Trauma Association (n.d.) states that, in the UK alone, it is estimated that 10,000 women a year may experience PTSD as a result of a traumatic birth, and a further 200,000 may feel traumatized and develop some symptoms. However, the study into the impact of traumatic birth is a relatively new area for research; consequently the amount of qualitative research available is moderate. I, therefore, hope that my study will add value to the current research discussion. I also anticipated that the insight gained from this research would be enlightening and helpful for my own counselling practice, and the wider counselling community. Given the magnitude of the problem, there is a high probability that Counsellors will encounter clients who have suffered a traumatic birth. This is therefore a useful piece of research for any Counsellor to read. I hope that Counsellors who do so will gain valuable insight which will broaden their understanding, sensitivity and empathy.

What the literature says

A search of the literature resulted in papers predominantly focusing on Post-Traumatic Stress Disorder (PTSD) and subsyndromal Post-Traumatic Stress Symptoms (PTSS). The majority of the papers focused on incidence and causal factors. As this research focuses on the impact, it was decided that information on causal factors would be outside the focus of this review. None of my participants were diagnosed with, nor tested for, PTSD, although some described symptoms which matched PTSS. It may therefore have seemed fitting to concentrate on literature which focused on PTSS. However, there is much controversy regarding the subjective nature of the diagnosis of PTSD (White et al. 2006), and the results of this literature review revealed divergence between researchers with regards to the measures used for classification of PTSD. There is therefore some doubt over whether women in some of the studies meet the diagnostic criteria for PTSD (Olde et al. 2006; Alcorn et al. 2010). Given the nature of this research, and the fact that post-traumatic stress is experienced on a continuum anyway, it seemed appropriate to review papers regardless of their focus on PTSD or PTSS. The following review should be taken in the context that many women who are subject to a traumatic birth will not experience PTSD or PTSS. The trauma may nevertheless have an impact on their lives.

PTSD was given formal recognition in DSM-III in 1980, and was defined as an anxiety disorder resulting from exposure to extreme events which were outside of the normal human experience (American Psychiatric Association, 1980). Given that the initial research work on PTSD came from the study of Vietnam War veterans, it is understandable that the nature of these extreme events was on the scale of war, natural and man-made disasters, rape and torture. Childbirth would not be recognized in this classification, because it is a normal event for approximately half of the population (Olde et al. 2006). In 1994, there was a change in criteria. DSM-IV (American Psychiatric Association, 1994) criteria stated a person has to have experienced, or witnessed, an incident which involved actual, or threatened, death, or serious injury, and that person's response is intense fear, helplessness or horror. This of course could describe what some women experience in childbirth.

Interest in birth as a traumatic event began to take hold in the mid-1990s as case reports emerged of women experiencing PTSD symptoms following childbirth (Ballard et al. 1995; Fones 1996). A quantitative study by Wijma et al. (1997), and a qualitative study by Allen (1998), were the first of a series of studies examining prevalence and predictors, which seemed to be the focus of research for the next ten years. More recently, research has started to look at the longer term implications of birth trauma, such as relationships with partners; mother–child relationships, and the impact on future childbearing. At about the same time as the interest in birth trauma arose, another area of trauma began to raise its profile. Traditionally, the emphasis in trauma research has focused on adverse medical, psychological and societal effects. In the 1990s, interest also turned to the positive changes that could occur following trauma. Whilst this has been given a number of labels, the term Post-Traumatic Growth (PTG) became the most prevalent. Initially PTG was recognized as a result of traumatic events such as combat; more recently PTG has been identified following numerous different traumatic events, suggesting that PTG is a result of the subjective experience of the event, rather than the type of event (Linley and Joseph 2004). In a systematic review of thirty-nine studies, Linley and Joseph (2004) asserted that positive change is commonly reported in around 30–70% of survivors of various traumatic events.

It is not necessarily the nature of the birth, but the woman's perception of the birth, which makes it traumatic (Allen 1998; Creedy et al. 2000; Beck 2004a). Fear, pain, being out of control, having no say in the birth, concern for the baby, and perceived poor care, are some of the factors which give rise to birth trauma. This can have an impact on how a woman sees herself and her place in the world. Women may see themselves differently, a shadow of their former selves, feeling they have failed at something for which their body was built. The realization that something so appalling can happen and that they cannot control it, may mean their world is no longer a safe place. Afterwards, some women report feeling fear, frustration, guilt (Souza et al. 2009), anger and anxiety (Beck 2004b) and depression (Ballard et al. 1995; Beck 2004b; Hofberg and Brockington 2000). Some women experience flashbacks and nightmares, which Beck (2004b) likens to a movie of their trauma. There may be a numbing of self, detachment (Ayers et al. 2006; Beck 2004b) and actual dissociation (Beck 2004b). However, PTSS is not experienced by all women who experience a traumatic birth. It would be useful to compare thoughts, emotions and cognitive processing of women who experience PTSS, with those who do not. A study by Ayers (2007) examined this subject. Themes of the birth experience as one of panic, anger, thoughts of death, mental defeat and dissociation, were reported predominantly by women with PTSS. Women without PTSS reported thinking about the baby, making decisions about the labour, and reported more positive emotions in response to their own actions. After birth, women with PTSS reported more painful memories, intrusive thoughts and rumination. However, women without symptoms tended to focus on the present and benefits, such as their baby, the improvement in their health, and the meaning of the birth for others. The processes adopted by the women without symptoms showed a tendency to find purpose or meaning in their life. This is one of the primary strategies in the rebuilding of assumptive worlds noted by Janoff-Bulman (2004). Both groups said they tried to avoid thinking about the birth; this is noteworthy given that avoidance is normally associated as a symptom of PTSD.

Mother–infant attachment problems have been found as a result of birth trauma (Fones 1996; Allen 1998; Ballard et al. 1995; Beck 2004b; Ayers et al. 2006; Soet et al. 2003; Nichols and Ayers 2007; Souza et al. 2009). Bailham and Joseph (2003) speculate that problems with bonding may be a result of avoidance, hyper-vigilance and numbing. To the avoidant mother, the child may be a constant reminder of the trauma, and may cause a re-experiencing of the event. A hyper-vigilant mother may become more anxious, or irritable, with her child. In the case of a mother suffering from emotional numbing, a lack of interaction and emotional responsiveness to the baby could result. In a qualitative study, Ayers et al. (2006) found the mother–baby bond was affected, with mothers reporting initial feelings of rejection towards the baby. Most women reported that feelings for their child did develop over time, although this might have taken between one and five years, whilst a few women reported ongoing difficulty in the relationship. Women reported either avoidant, or overprotective, behaviour towards their baby. A study by Nichols and Ayers (2007) corroborated this, reporting either an avoidant/rejecting, or over-anxious/overprotecting, attachment pattern. Conversely in a quantitative study, Ayers et al. (2007a) found that PTSD was not related to the quality of the mother baby bond. The difference in findings may be because of the wording of the research, as the 2007 study looked at the behavioural aspects of bonding, i.e. was the baby taken care of, as opposed to the emotional aspects? Timing of the study may also have been an issue. The timing of the study was only nine weeks after birth, where it could be argued that the impact of PTSD was not yet apparent. Ayers et al. (2007a) also suggest the difference in results may be due to the difference in focus and levels of PTSD for the two types of study, with the qualitative study looking at clinically significant levels of PTSD and the quantitative looking at general stress responses.

In a more recent study, Elmir et al. (2011) researched the experience of early mothering by women who had undergone an emergency hysterectomy following childbirth. The mothers' operation forced a separation from their babies for lengthy periods. The mothers viewed this as a loss of precious bond forming time. The mother–baby bond suffered, which caused feelings of guilt, and of being a bad mother. Concern over who was looking after their baby, and distress that other family members had seen and held their baby first, was also reported. Some mothers felt guilt, and a sense of failure, for the perceived distress and trauma they had put their babies through. For many mothers, breastfeeding was seen as a way of undoing their initial failure and of acquiring the maternal role; an inability to do so because of the trauma their body has suffered was experienced as failure and shame. The significance of breastfeeding was examined in Beck and Watson's (2008) study of the impact of trauma on breastfeeding. They found that women wanted to prove themselves as mothers, and atone for the baby's traumatic arrival. Successful breastfeeding was healing, as it helped women to regain self-esteem, confidence, and restored faith in their bodies. Sadly, for other women, breastfeeding was not such a positive experience. For some, the physical injuries made it a painful ordeal, whilst trauma to their body sometimes resulted in insufficient milk supply. Frightening flashbacks were reported. For some women, it was another invasion and violation of their body and, for some, breastfeeding was an empty affair which only drew attention to the detachment they felt from their babies. This detached feeling, and subsequent behaviour, has also been viewed in depressed women who may be less responsive, communicative and in tune with their babies (Field et al. 1990).

Bowlby's (1973) attachment theory highlights the importance of mother–baby attachment for the child's development and emotional health. The literature search found gaps in research on the long-term impact on children of mothers with PTSD and PTSS. However, research is available for mothers with depression. The detrimental impact on the children has been noted as an increased risk of social deficits, affective disorders, behavioural problems, achievement deficits and adjustment difficulties (Anderson and Hammen 1993; Cogill et al. 1986; Murray et al. 1996).

Traumatic birth can also have an impact on the woman's relationship with her partner (Fones 1996; Allen 1998; Parfitt and Ayers 2009; Nichols and Ayers 2007). In a qualitative study by Ayers et al. (2006), the themes of support and strain on the relationship emerged. Even good support offered by partners was reported as just not enough to heal the distress. All participants reported strain on their relationship, either as a result of loss of self-esteem because of the birth, loss of sexual intimacy, disagreements about the birth, women blaming men for the events of the birth, and women not giving partners time or attention. Conversely, in a quantitative study, Ayers et al. (2007b) found that PTSD symptoms were not related to the marital relationship in mothers who reported severe PTSD nine weeks after birth. However, it could be that nine weeks post birth may be too short a period of time to truly measure the impact on relationships. The difference in results may be due to the difference in focus and levels of PTSD for the two types of study; with the qualitative study looking at clinically significant levels of PTSD, and the quantitative looking at general stress responses (Ayers et al. 2007b). One should also be careful of drawing any generalizations from qualitative studies. Research reports that sexual dysfunction had an impact on relationships (O'Driscoll 1994; Allen 1998; Ayers et al. 2006). Nichols and Ayers (2007) found women avoided sex because it was a reminder of the trauma, they wanted to protect their battered body, or through a fear of pregnancy.

The fear of future childbirth has a huge impact on many. Hofberg and Brockington's (2000) study of women with secondary tokophobia (fear of childbirth as a result of a traumatic birth), found that when two of their participants suffered miscarriages, and one an ectopic pregnancy, the women expressed enormous relief that the pregnancies did not result in delivery. The fear was so great for one woman, that she underwent a termination. Nine out of eleven women in their sample arranged elective caesarean sections. This desire for elective caesarean sections as a result of previous birth trauma is corroborated in studies by Ryding et al. (1998). This obviously has a significant, ongoing, impact on medical resources and the physical recovery of the mother. However, Hofberg and Brockington (2000) found that women who received their preferred birth method fared better psychologically than those who did not. Beck and Watson (2010) looked at subsequent childbirth following a traumatic childbirth. In a study of thirty-five women, they found women described feelings of fear, terror anxiety, panic, dread and denial during their subsequent pregnancy. Women developed strategies, such as making detailed plans to rectify things that had gone wrong previously. Three quarters of the women found a subsequent birth to be a better experience; for some it was healing and empowering, but sadly, for some, the second birth was not healing because it was also traumatic, or because the hurt from the first birth was too huge to forget. The potential healing nature of subsequent birth is also found in Thomson and Downe's (2010) qualitative study. The theme 'Changing the future to change the past' is reflective of the redemptive, healing and transformational nature of sub-sequent positive birthing experience. Thomson and Downe (2010) report that the joy that was experienced, allowed the women to reframe and re-integrate their beliefs surrounding their birth trauma. However, the trauma was forgiven rather than forgotten, as a number of women felt the trauma had still left scars. Unfortunately, the story was different for women who did not conceive again; unable to internalize their trauma, they continued to experience a continuation of recall and flashbacks. Ayers et al. (2006) reported that women who did not conceive again experienced a sense of loss for the children they had wanted but would not have.

Post-Traumatic Growth (PTG) is described by Calhoun and Tedeschi (1998, 2000) as a positive change in either beliefs or functioning that can be experienced as a result of the struggle with a major loss or trauma. Their Functional Descriptive Model of PTG likens the process to that of an earthquake, with the trauma being a seismic event that threatens many of the schematic structures that have guided the individual's beliefs and actions. PTG arises from the individual's cognitive struggle to resolve this challenge to their assumptive world, which is worked through by a process of automatic, then deliberate, rumination. This results in a development of new schemas. Joseph and Linley's (2005) organismic valuing model of PTG is also concerned with changes in assumptive worlds but this theory has its roots in Person-Centred theory. It argues that individuals, guided by their innate tendency towards actualization, have a basic propensity to rebuild their assumptive worlds. As such, PTG is not a qualitatively different experience that is distinct from other normal human development, but is rather a natural lifespan developmental event (Joseph and Linley 2008). Inherent in the concept of PTG is that individual levels of psychological development have undergone a change beyond pre-trauma levels. Therefore, PTG is not the same as coping, or resilience, which are concerned with endurance or returning to previous levels of functioning (McGrath and Linley 2006). Tedeschi, Park and Calhoun (1998) categorize five outcomes of PTG: increased appreciation of life, sense of new possibilities in life, increased personal strength, improvement in close relationships, and positive spiritual change. Not everyone experiences PTG, therefore the model emphasizes the importance of pre-trauma variables (such as personality and previous trauma); event related variables (for example severity) and post event variables (such as social support and amount of distress) (Sawyer et al. 2012). The existence of PTG is not without its detractors. McFarland and Alvaro (2000) ascertain that individuals may be motivated to cope with trauma by perceiving a personal growth that does not reflect the reality. Reporting the positive may ease some of the distress. Taylor et al. (2000) used the term *positive illusions* which may correlate to denial and longer term poor psychological outcomes. There is also considerable debate about the effectiveness of the tools used to measure PTG, as most rely on the subjective perception of growth (Ford et al.

2008). However Joseph and Butler (2010), in noting the limitations of retrospection, note that positive change has been measured through other means.

My search criteria could not locate any published studies specifically examining PTG following traumatic childbirth. However, my search identified two studies examining 'Growth' after childbirth (Sawyers and Ayers 2009, 2012). Whilst neither study throws much light on the link between traumatic birth and PTG (although this was not their primary aim), the second study is perhaps the most useful as it found that women who had a caesarean section displayed higher levels of growth in comparison to women who had a normal vaginal delivery. The authors ascertain that obstetric intervention may be viewed as a more stressful delivery experience, and that the findings are therefore consistent with the view that more severe events stimulate greater growth. However, there is a contradiction in that they also found participants' subjective rating of the birth as traumatic, was not significantly related to growth. There are a number of limitations to this study. Firstly the mean PTSD score after birth was low, which hinders understanding of the relationship between traumatic stress symptoms and PTG. Secondly the author's analysis indicated that non-respondents were more likely to have suffered from higher levels of psychological distress and therefore their sample was probably under-represented by women who had found birth distressing. Finally, the assessment of growth was carried out only eight weeks after the birth which is probably too soon after the event for PTG to occur (Joseph and Linley 2005; Tedeschi et al. 2004). Souza et al. (2009), in a study of Maternal Near-Miss Syndrome, found that despite great suffering, most women managed to find something positive in the experience. For some, it was a wake up call as to who, and what, was important in life; to some it was a reappraisal of their relationship with God and a change to give more value to God-given things rather than material possessions; the transitory nature of life had become all too obvious, and for some this had a direct impact on how they took care of themselves in future. However, this study was carried out before hospital discharge when the traumatic experience was still raw. So, it is not known whether this was long-lived.

Participants

For the purposes of my research, I took the view that the birth trauma should be self-defined, reasoning this would attract diverse participation, and that maximum variation sampling would offer further insight. As my aim was to gather detailed information, purposive sampling was utilized (Smith et al. 2009), by selecting female, qualified Counsellors who had experienced a traumatic birth and were willing to verbalize their experience. Counsellors, experienced in personal development, and sharing thoughts and feelings in-depth may have offered a richer depth of awareness and language than I might otherwise have encountered.

My selection criteria for inclusion were women who:

- Had experienced a self-defined traumatic birth which resulted in the birth of a robust, live, child.
- Were qualified practising Counsellors, qualified to a minimum of diploma level.
- Had access to supervision to ensure that they had the necessary support.
- Had access to personal counselling.

- Considered themselves to be grounded in their experience and able to discuss the impact without negative repercussions.

My decision was to exclude Counsellors:

- Whose traumatic birth experience was less than five years ago.
- Were currently undergoing counselling as a repercussion of the trauma.
- Were pregnant.
- Were known to me.

The criteria allowed the sample to be purposeful, but were wide enough to allow variability in factors such as age, time elapsed from the birth, cause, societal factors and experience. In order to recruit participants, advertisements were placed with Therapy Today and BACP Research online notice-boards. A poster was placed in local universities, colleges and thirty counselling agencies in the North West of England. In order to add to triangulation, participants were invited to bring any diaries, poetry, photographs or items which could enlighten their experience. The planned sample size was between four and six participants; a practical consideration given the timescale as a larger sample size might have hindered my ability to fully immerse myself in the experience of my participants. All women were of white British descent. At the time of the study, all women were aged in their mid to late forties. The interval between their traumatic birth and this study was between fifteen and twenty-five years.

Three women experienced assisted vaginal deliveries (ventouse and/or forceps), with tearing and/or episiotomies requiring stitches. Two of the three women have experienced ongoing physical repercussions. For one participant, the trauma occurred immediately post-partum in the form of a potentially life-threatening condition resulting in a six-week recovery period. This was the first child for all participants. Two women went on to have one more child, both with a five year gap between children (Joanne and Diane). Both of these second births were difficult, with Diane describing her second birth as traumatic too. One woman (Alex) had two further children. Both births contained considerable risk and difficulty, although she did not categorize them as traumatic. One woman (Sandy) went on to have three more children and all were uncomplicated births.

Data collection

In line with my research philosophy and phenomenological approach, I decided to use semi-structured, face-to-face, recorded interviews as a data collection method, based on the following questions:

- What were the expectations of childbirth? (i.e. thoughts, feelings – what brought them about?)
- Although this research is really looking at the impact of your traumatic birth it would be useful to briefly describe the birth and what went wrong for you. Can you remember your thoughts and feelings at the time? What were you feelings about yourself? How did you cope?
- Can you describe the impact on your relationships? (i.e. with your husband/partner, with your baby, with parents or others that you are close to? Thoughts/ feelings about how it impacted?)
- What was the impact on your relationship with friends, particularly those who had just given birth themselves or were due to?

- How did it impact on your decision to have other children? (How does that make you feel now?)
- How have your thoughts/feelings changed in the time elapsed?
- Did anything good come out of this trauma – post-traumatic growth?
- How is it for you now talking about this?
- Is there anything that you would like to add – are there other areas not covered upon which your experience had an impact?

Findings

After analysing the data using IPA methodology (Smith et al. 2009), the following master themes and sub-themes were identified (see Table 9).

Master theme 1: Processing the Trauma

Sub-theme 1.1: Dissociation as a coping mechanism: Whilst all women experience pain, fear and loss of control, three of the four women described their birth trauma in relatively factual, as opposed to emotional, terms. These women also showed dissociation at the time of the trauma. Emotionally, they had removed themselves to a safer place. Alex described it as: *"I felt like I was floating somewhere else ... I felt like it wasn't happening to me. Like it was really happening to someone else. And yet I knew exactly what was going on".* Diane stated, *"I was worried and everything but I was more in a bubble than anything, I don't think it was impacting on me as I would have expected ... I can see myself in that situation but it was almost like I was observing what was going on rather than so much experiencing it, you know".* Joanne could not recall her feelings at the time of the trauma: *"I can't remember because I squidged it out".* In contrast, Sandy described her traumatic birth with

Master themes	1 - Processing the Trauma	2 - Sense of Self	3 - Family Relationships
Sub-themes	1.1 Dissociation as a coping mechanism	2.1 Loss	3.1 Marital relationships
	1.2 The baby as meaning- maker	2.2 Seeking redemption	3.2 Mother– baby relationship
	1.3 Keeping quiet and trying to cope	2.3 Reassertion	3.3 Future pregnancies
	1.4 Working through depression	2.4 Post-traumatic growth	
	1.5 Putting the bad to good use		

Table 9. Master and sub-themes.

great emotion. She did not mention dissociative indicators: *"It's scary. I think it's the scariness of it, not being in control, not knowing what to do, not being listened to, not being helped, not being understood ... That pain I will never forget it ever, ever ... If I could erase it from my mind I would really like to"*.

Sub-theme 1.2: The baby as meaning-maker: The delivery of a healthy baby was central to their processing and the sense-making of their experience. In the immediate aftermath of the trauma, some of the women described concentrating on the needs of the baby rather than ruminating on their own misfortune. As a potentially life-threatening condition developed in her body, Alex recalls the focus was on taking care of her baby: *"And all I could think of was 'I haven't fed this baby properly and I was focused on that. I must feed this baby'"*. For Alex, the trauma was not forgotten, but it was pushed to the background: *"I was certainly aware that, all of a sudden, I had gone through a massive trauma, and this massive life event, and yet I still had this baby. I had to look after her"*. Diane's account was similar: *"And then he was born and you have a baby then haven't you. I had to stay in hospital for about six days. And he was a bit jaundiced. So I think straight after the birth I was more focused on him"*. Joanne seemed to find meaning by balancing the trauma against the outcome of a healthy baby: *"I was upset that it had happened but okay because my baby was strong and well ... So I think the saving grace through all of it was that she was totally okay"*. For Sandy, her baby provided all the meaning she needed, she could concentrate on the positive and he became her healing agent: *"Giving birth is not easy and mine was particularly traumatic but you come out with something at the end. With a lot of other traumas, like soldiers coming back from Afghanistan without limbs, they have not got anything to show for their trauma, they have had things taken away from them. Whereas the difference with a birth and giving birth to a baby that's perfectly healthy, at least you have got that baby to help the wounds heal I think"*. Sandy movingly affirmed that despite everything: *"I still managed to give birth to a perfectly healthy baby boy, so I think that's what heals. It's him"*.

Sub-theme 1.3: Keeping quiet and trying to cope: In the aftermath of the trauma, none of the participants talked to anybody, neither family or friends, nor professionals, about their experience and how it had left them feeling. Their process was to keep quiet, suppress emotions, and try to cope. Rumination was not part of their process at this stage. For Alex, it appeared safer to keep quiet than to face what had happened: *"I don't think I had quite worked out what was happening to me. I don't think I quite knew. I couldn't articulate it to myself. You know that fear, that 'Oh God, I could have died' and 'This wasn't quite perfect'. I don't think I had quite processed it. I* *wouldn't have known what to say to people ... I think I was downplaying it to myself to survive and underplaying it to people actually. Because if I really admitted how awful it was I might suddenly feel it".* Joanne was silent and suppressed her emotions by keeping busy: *"The coping was suppressing the emotions. I literally put a lid on it, you don't go there. And so I just went into the practical side of caring for a new baby and doing as much as I could and gradually building it back up and putting up with the discomfort and pain".* Diane described how she coped in the aftermath: *"You pick yourself up, you get on with life. I don't think I ever really talked about what it was like ... It is an experience that has been boxed off".* Diane's silence was so contained that even her husband was unaware that she felt her birth was traumatic: *"When I said to my husband that I was going to do this* [i.e. the research into the impact of traumatic birth], *he said to me is that a traumatic birth?"* Sandy also decided to seal the experience away: *"I didn't talk about the labour ... I've never told anyone how I felt ... I think I shut it away in a little box".*

Sub-theme 1.4: Working through depression: All of the women experienced what they now term as depression, although they may not have recognized it at the time. For Diane the depression emerged as she returned home following the birth. For Alex and Joanne depression occurred after later births, although both attribute it to their earlier birth trauma. Sandy's experience was different as whilst she suffered from Post-Natal Depression (PND) after the birth of her last child, she believes this was a hormone imbalance rather than a belated repercussion of her trauma. Alex, Joanne and Diane sought different methods of support to work through their depression. After her third birth, which was difficult if not perilous and traumatic, Alex described her feelings as: *"I just remember suddenly feeling this awful panic and felt clammy and just thinking 'oh it's not fair, it's just not fair'… And just feeling really, really low for about eight weeks. So low I couldn't, didn't want to go out. I had got through the other two quite stoically but with this one I didn't have anything left".* Having the support of her husband, mother and a close friend she felt held enough to explore and ruminate on herself and this new murky world: *"I'd gone right down but I thought you know what, I am okay. I'm still here. And this is about as bad as it could have got. I can do this. I can even do this misery. If it carries on I can do it. And that for me was like feeling the pain and doing it anyway. And realising what my boundaries, you know I touched my edges and I was okay. I'd stopped frightening myself. I worked out that I was able and I was strong. What I was able to cope with. I sort of processed the fear".*

Joanne recollects little of her depression but remembers a number of factors which combined to threaten her resilience, resulting in: *"I was finding it difficult to cope. I think deep down it was the trauma coming out".* Joanne sought medical help and was referred to a psychologist for hypnosis. Diane described her depression: *"If I had had a couple of days which were good I would think oh something is going to happen now, you know. Tiredness and lack of motivation, I think that was the main thing and just not being able to keep on top of everything; everything seemed to pile up. Everything seemed an effort".* Diane attended a support group to help a friend but found it valuable for her own process of making sense of her feelings: *"I never even considered it was depression. I was going to a support group and any arguments I had with my husband or anything I would say oh horrible day today, tell everybody about it you know and apply the 12-step programme to it. I was very, very lucky".*

Sub-theme 1.5: Putting the bad to good use: The ability to help others brought some meaning to their traumatic experience. Alex recounted how her decision to become a Counsellor was a direct result of her experience: *"So that really helped to shape me wanting to get into counselling. Also what isn't okay to say, when people say the wrong things. How damaging that is, I know that. I've learnt what not to do, what not to say. I think I'm pretty bloody good at helping people now because I have been there"*. Joanne described a similar desire. In her case she has developed an affinity to working with women: *"I realised that it (counselling) brought everything together, it was basically what I wanted to do, to help people get over things ... Some energy is out there that I would rather work with women and actually I now specifically state I work with women"*. Sandy explained her motivation for agreeing to this research: *"If I can help I will talk my heart out"*.

Master theme 2: Sense of Self
Sub-theme 2.1: Loss: All women experienced a sense of loss because of the nature of the birth and its aftermath. This was more than a grieving for a beautiful reaffirming birth experience. This was a sense that part of their very being had been lost too. Alex suffered PND, and describes the shock in facing up to her new self: *"Oh my God, I can't believe I was anxious, I'm not an anxious person! I've never experienced anything like that before, you know. I coped. I don't do depression. You know I'm not really the anxious type. You know I'm dead healthy. You know. Well rounded. You know ... that was my self-image. Not exactly invulnerable, but strong. I've got a lovely family. I'm not going to get things like that. Nothing awful has really happened to me. So I think in the first year after my baby was born I had to re-evaluate who I was"*. Five years after the birth, a series of factors culminated in a referral to a psychologist.

Joanne explained how she now viewed herself: *"It's failure ... you failed to have a normal birth and you have failed to be the perfect Mum and you failed this and you failed that, you are not good enough".* In addition to her sense of failure Joanne also described a detachment and loss from her womanhood: *"I associate sex with pain and the pelvic area with pain and discomfort … I was denying parts of myself. I was denying my womb space really because the whole thing, you know the woman thing, has just got pain associated with it".* Some twenty years after the birth, Joanne recently attended a retreat and: *"I am now looking at my sort of pelvic area in a different light now and actually healing it … It's amazing, that psychological reprogramming to honour that part of my womanhood if you like which I have denied".* Sandy revealed an utter sense of shock in her inability to control either her own body or the circumstances of the birth. She too saw herself as a failure: *"My first birth was completely out of control, I wasn't in control, you've never done it before, you don't know what to expect but I was not expecting not to be able to catch my breath, not to be able to do it. I suppose I was almost annoyed with myself that thousands of others can. What is wrong with me, why can't I do this, lots of people can, why can't I?".* A theme that Sandy returned to on three occasions was that during her traumatic birth nobody seemed to listen to her, that she was not important. The traumatic nature of the birth and her treatment shook her confidence in the safety of the world and her place in it: *"It was as if I didn't matter. And that was scary. It's the first time I have ever felt like that. It just felt like I was the vessel and the baby was the most important thing, you know bringing this child into the world healthy which was the main thing which of course it is. But at what cost? At what cost!?".*

Sub-theme 2.2: Seeking redemption: All four women breastfed their babies, although their physical condition made this difficult. This seemed to fulfil a number of functions, for whilst it gave their baby the best start in life, it also helped re-establish some control and claw back some self-esteem and sense of normality. There was a redemptive element in this breastfeeding, as it asserted their status as successful nurturing mothers. Alex stated: *"I had all the obstacles* (for breastfeeding), *mastitis, terrible mastalgia, you know really painful feeding. And I still kept going. I couldn't control anything else and I was so out of control with everything else. I had no control over my childbirths. It was the one thing I could do".* Joanne said: *"I needed the control and to get back, be normal … I was limited in what I could do. Just lying there and feeding my baby, in I was doing something I could do".* Sandy described it as: *"I was going to breastfeed … yeah, I wanted to be a real mum a proper mum".* Diane stated: *"I would have been really devastated if I couldn't have breast fed. …* [It was important] *in getting close to your baby and nurturing your baby".*

Sub-theme 2.3: Reassertion: Joanne, Sandy and Diane believed they had put themselves in the hands of experts, had been too compliant and had been let down. Armed with a better understanding of their body in labour, they resolved not to allow this to happen for their second birth. The second births demonstrated an internal locus of evaluation not apparent in their first births. Talking of her preparation for her second birth Sandy said: *"It gave me the strength to go into my later labours knowing that I wouldn't just leave myself in their hands again, I wouldn't take their word for what was going on all the time. I wouldn't just accept what people say anymore. I would question it … I would not be a martyr … So I put myself in control".* On being advised that her second baby might need to be induced, Joanne was able to assert herself and take more control of her pain relief: *"I was quite happy to scream I want the epidural now! They didn't catheterise me so much because I was able to explain and they were really understanding".* Diane explained her view of herself in her first birth: *"I was like a frightened rabbit the first time".* In preparation for her second birth, she decided: *"I am going to be able to express myself and say what I need"*. In actuality, she did listen to her internal locus of evaluation. During her second labour, the hospital wanted to send her home deeming she was not yet in labour, whilst she believed she was: *"But I didn't go because I knew I could feel my body and I knew what was happening and even if there were authoritative people who were saying no you're not, I was more assertive and said no"*.

Sub-theme 2.4: Post-traumatic growth: Three participants believed their trauma had resulted in post-traumatic growth. However, this is not to say that their suffering and their journey was forgotten or forgiven. Nor that the growth compensates for the suffering encountered. A number of the women commented on the duality of their journey. Alex explained an increased awareness of self: *"I knew where my edges were. Knowing that I could go quite a long way out of my things going wrong range. I could go way out. They could all go horribly wrong and I wasn't going to disintegrate. I nearly did but I didn't ... It's made me nicer. Probably a bit easier to be with. And it has made it easier for people to be vulnerable with me. More open to I think. Softer ... [but] I have regret for that peri-natal period. I would have liked to enjoy them more as babies and I feel sad that I didn't ... it traumatized me and the effects have stayed with me ever since. Good and bad. Since then I've been more easily triggered in anxiety provoking situations"*.

Diane stated: *"I think it was a strength that I felt more at one with myself, you know that I was able and capable ... I think it certainly helped me develop as a person ... [but sadly] not wanting any more children, that is probably the most dramatic impact [of the traumatic birth]"*. Joanne said: *"It has made me who I am, it has made me stronger in some ways ... it gave me some belief in my-self. You know if you can get through this you can get through anything"*. But Joanne also tragically experienced ongoing *"guilt that my daughter thought I blamed her for my medical problems"*. Sandy felt differently. Whilst she recognized she was more assertive in her later births, she saw this as a particular circumstance and did not relate this to growth. She was vehement that: *"Nothing good came out of that labour. Only my baby"*.

Master theme 3: Family Relationships

Sub-theme 3.1: Marital relationships: The birth trauma had an impact on marital relationships. Sandy and Diane felt very let down by their husbands for not protecting them during their birth trauma. Experiencing anger and hurt, they took refuge in their baby, pushing their husband aside. This anger had been forgotten over time but their reaction in recalling this was very emotional. Sandy said: *"I would look at my husband when I was going through this as if to say please save me, do something ... [and] I did hold it against him for not sticking up for me. I remember us having a row and me saying you never fight my corner, you weren't there for me in that labour. And that really hurt him. I probably did shut him [her husband] out a bit because he [her baby] was mine and I was not sharing. You have no idea what I went through to get this child, he is all mine"*.

Diane talked, not only of her anger, but of how the birth had not been the unifying experience that she had anticipated: *"I was angry with him that he wasn't more in control of the situation. It was like you know you were supposed to be looking after me and all this went on ... He was part of the birth but wasn't ... There was definitely a dramatic effect on our relationship but I felt that my husband had been very much babied by me, when I was giving my attention to a baby he was sort of like whoah"*. Conversely, Alex and Joanne both felt supported. Joanne talked of support and protection: *"There is relief that he had been there supporting me but also guilt that he had to see me go through* that. *After the birth of our second child he was adamant that we were not going through that again. He was not putting me through that again*". Alex described their relationship as she suffered the depths of depression following her third birth: "*I said I can't cope. So he had to … I always knew he was solid and there for me. So I think I recognised how strong he was. And then I think that when I started to recover myself, he recognised my strength as well. … There were loads of stresses in our relationship that had come in but ultimately it brought us closer together. You know we were, we took over when each one needed it*".

Sub-theme 3.2: Mother–baby relationship: Bonding with their baby was a source of discussion for all participants. Only one participant, Sandy, felt an instant love and adoration. This love was all consuming. "*I really went into mum mode. I would lose days because I would just sit in pjs with my baby, just me and him. It was gorgeous, it was great … It became all encompassing. I couldn't leave my baby with even my husband on his own, he was mine, it was really all on*". For the other participants, there appears to be something missing from the early description of motherhood. Two of the participants show this in their hesitancy in their description of bonding. Joanne stated: "*It probably did affect the bonding, probably more than I give it credit for or actually would care to remember*". Diane seemed unsure and raised the issue of difficulty in breastfeeding, suggesting it may have had an impact on that initial bond: "*I think I bonded well with my son … [*but*] I didn't think what a gorgeous baby or anything. We did have difficulty with breastfeeding at first*". Alex was very clear about how she bonded with all three of her children. On her first child following her birth trauma, she recalls: "*I didn't really bond. I just stared at this child and remember thinking, I can't manage this*". Alex thought the impact of her trauma materialized after her third birth. She did not initially bond with her baby.

And then: *"I just remember feeling a rush of love. I just remember going Oh my God I love you. I'm so ... and I was thinking why did I have this third baby up until then. And then I realised, I do want her"*. Feeling guilty for not initially bonding and trying to compensate for her depression: *"I held her all the time, I didn't put her down for those weeks. I think I felt bad for how numb I was, how anxious I was. I held her all the time. I fed her all the time. I wouldn't let her out of my sight"*.

Sub-theme 3.3: Future pregnancies: The trauma left all women very fearful of future pregnancies, but this was overridden by the desire for a family and a common belief that it could not happen again. Happily, a redemptive birth gave Sandy the confidence to go on to have the large family she longed for. Sandy stated: *"Well I sort of reconciled myself to the fact that it couldn't be any worse and I felt everything that could go wrong had gone wrong. ... but every now and again, the first birth would come back to haunt me. As I entered hospital to have (second child) I was as sick as a dog through nerves. ... She was a darling [her second baby], two-hour labour, I could never thank her enough"*. Sadly for Joanne and Diane, difficult second births brought their childbearing years to a premature end. Joanne said: *"There was fear of going through it again but it also felt right having a second child and the thought that it is not going to happen twice like that"*. Her second birth was problematic and the decision was made that Joanne's husband would be sterilized. *"It wasn't worth the risk of me getting pregnant again"*. Physical and psychological injuries from Diane's first birth impacted on her readiness to have another child: *"I had a lot of stitches and things, so physically I was not going to go for another baby very quickly. ... and also because of the depression afterwards. I think it was a long time before one, I thought I could go through birth again and two that I could cope with another baby again. ... I thought the second one is not going to be as bad"*. After a traumatic second birth, Diane decided: *"... this is not happening ever again. A few years later my husband said it would be nice to have another baby and I said no thanks. Oh no ... I wouldn't put myself through that again"*. For Diane, the premature end of her childbearing years was the most significant impact of her birth trauma: *"Not wanting any more children, that is probably the most dramatic impact* [of the traumatic birth]*"*.

Discussion

This phenomenological study exploring the impact of traumatic birth identified three master themes: Processing the Trauma; Sense of Self; and Family Relationships. There is considerable overlap in these areas, with one often impacting on the other. For example, the subordinate theme 'post-traumatic growth' could arguably have been categorized within the 'Processing the Trauma' theme. However, as three of my participants tended to talk of PTG in terms of their sense of self, as opposed to the process of how they gained that growth, it seemed more appropriate to categorize it as such.

The first category identified the women's process and sense making of the trauma. All women described emotions of pain, fear, powerlessness and loss of control during the birth. Three of the women described their reaction to the unfolding trauma itself as one of dissociation: *"I felt like it wasn't happening to me. Like it was really happening to someone else"*. (Alex). Dissociation at the time of the birth shielded them from a horrific reality. Dissociation is a controversial subject. It can be seen as a normal protective process, whereby a person disconnects from parts of an experience in order to prevent being overwhelmed (Etherington 2003), or as Nijenhuis et al. (2001) suggest, a failure of the normal integrative mental process. But dissociation is not a perfect answer, and may have negative side effects, for example nightmares, flashbacks or emotional numbing (Etherington 2003). This numbing effect was experienced by Diane, who noted how she spoke of her birth very factually, almost as if there was no emotional involvement there. The existence of negative emotions and dissociation in childbirth in this study correlates with other research (e.g. Olde et al. 2006; Creedy et al. 2000; Ayers 2007).

The safe arrival of their baby was a major part of the sense-making for all mothers. Mothers showed concern for the safety of their baby during the birth trauma, and afterwards they focused on the baby, rather than their own emotional and physical health. This focus was there irrespective of whether they felt an immediate bond with their baby or not. For Sandy, her baby was very clearly the meaning-maker of her trauma. She made the point that no matter how bad the birth was, no matter how much of a failure she had been, she had still given birth to a healthy baby who had healed her. She poignantly compared her birth trauma to military amputees, making the point that ultimately she had gained where they had only lost. Tennen and Affleck (2002) view this focus on the positive outcome as a meaning-making coping strategy, which in effect modifies the meaning of the trauma. The same type of cognitive processing was found in a study by Ayers (2007), where women retrospectively gave a more positive meaning to the experience by focusing on the baby. Ayers (2007) proposes that this process suggests all was worthwhile. However, Sandy's vehement assertion that nothing good came out of the trauma bar her son, highlights the complexity of this. The birth may well have been worthwhile, but that does not mean it was forgiven. Beck's (2004b) study of PTSD following a birth trauma, found her participants wanted to talk, talk, talk! A study of Brazilian women who experienced perilous births, found the women ruminating on the events (Souza et al. 2009). Conversely, a study by Ayers (2007) which compared women who had PTSS with those who did not, found neither group wanted to think about their trauma. The initial process of the women in this study was neither to think about, nor talk about, their birth. Two participants did not even share their thoughts with their husbands. So effective was Diane's secrecy that it was only when she announced she was to take part in this research, that her husband realized she had felt her birth was traumatic. This lack of communication between partners about the trauma was also noted in a Nichols and Ayers study (2007). Silence does have the potential to isolate, and both Alex and Joanne said that their social group of other mothers decreased in size. This could be detrimental when the company of other mothers can provide much support. The participants gave a complex web of reasons for the silence, for example it was their personality type to accept the cards dealt; the desire to put a lid on things and get on with it; the fear that people would not want to know; the fear that other people would not understand; that it might frighten others, especially mothers-to-be; and that they did not want to upset those close to them. These could be avoidant strategies, but it was only Alex who disclosed it as such: *"I think I was downplaying it to myself to survive and underplaying it to people actually. Because if I really admitted how awful it was I might suddenly feel it"*. All participants' birth traumas took place over fifteen years ago, but the research interview was the first time any of the women had ever talked about it in any detail. Following the interview all mentioned how good and therapeutic it had been to talk at last. Whilst it is outside the scope of this research, it seems plausible that the anonymity of today's social media, and the advent of sites discussing birth trauma, may make it easier for women to discuss their experiences without the fear of upsetting others or not being understood, factors which silenced some of this study's participants. In studies of PND in the general female population, Gavin et al. (2005) found 21% prevalence (cited in Wylie et al. 2011). All four of the women in this study experienced depression, with three directly relating it to their birth trauma. Whilst this qualitative study cannot be generalized, the high incidence of depression in this study is worthy of note. It is a sad statistic that self-harm is the main cause of maternal death in the first year post-partum (Wylie et al. 2011), and if birth trauma is a risk factor for depression, it should be noted by caregivers. Symptoms of PND and PTSD have some commonalities, for example sleep disturbance, trouble concentrating, avoidance, anger, guilt and shame. This brings into question the likelihood that some women will be misdiagnosed with PND, the more familiar condition, when PTSD may be more appropriate (White et al. 2006). Interestingly, the participants to this study did not label their emotions, or physiological symptoms, as PTS, but they did equate them to depression.

The mothers in this research worked through their depression in different ways: a support group (Diane), family support and rumination (Alex), and hypnosis (Joanne). Alex and Diane stressed how they worked through this, Alex *"touched my edges"* and *"processed the fear"* to come out the other side as stronger and more self-aware. Such gratifying triumph should not override the suffering of the women during this period. Alex poignantly talks about her depression, her shock at not recognizing herself and the loss of the initial bonding period with her child. Diane talks of the effort to get out of bed to change her baby's nappy and being overwhelmed by the most simple of tasks. There is little wonder that Beck (1999) described PND as a dangerous thief that causes misery and robs women of their time with their infants. The women's sense of self had been profoundly shaken as a result of the trauma. They equated their shock, being out of control, and their actions, with failure and a sense of weakness. They questioned why they could not do this properly when everyone else could. Joanne questioned whether she had done something wrong, equating her *"suffering"*, her *"pain"* with punishment (Joanne). Two of the women wondered whether they could trust themselves anymore, and questioned whether the birth had really been as bad as they thought. For Sandy, it appeared important that the extent of her pain had been validated by both an attending registrar, and later by her own doctor (Sandy). Despite the validation she questions whether she maybe has a low pain threshold and still blames herself for her failure (Sandy). Joanne was unsure whether the story in her head was true. Four years later, she had the opportunity to see her notes which reassured her she *"hadn't over-dramatized it"* (Joanne).

Their lack of control during labour was a recurring theme for all women, and correlates with findings in a number of studies (Allen 1998; Beck 2004b; Nichol and Ayers 2007). Etherington (2003) states that it is this helplessness which makes an event subjectively overwhelming; and that those who have some element of control, no matter how small, will fare better emotionally than those who feel helpless. Indeed the described helplessness links in with one of the DSM-IV criteria for PTSD, that the traumatic situation should involve fear, helplessness or horror. Breastfeeding gave the mothers an opportunity to reassert their control, give their baby the best start in life and to prove themselves in their new role. Despite their own physical condition, which made breastfeeding painful and difficult for some, and physiological reasons which could delay lactogenesis, all mothers in this study were determined to breastfeed in order to be a *"proper mum"* (Sandy). Of course, the stakes are high; success brings redress, fulfilment, and a closeness and pleasure in their baby. This closeness was described by Sandy as feeling like they were *"still connected"* (Sandy). This statement also suggests an element of protection and safety which perhaps she felt unable to provide during the birth trauma because she was not in control. Unfortunately, the redemptive possibility of breastfeeding was not to be experienced by all. Alex's resultant medical condition made breastfeeding excruciating, it took a while to establish and she recalls being *"really screwed up about that"* (Alex). However, her sense of achievement from eventually succeeding is shown in one of her closing comments *"They are all here, they're alive and they are gorgeous, healthy, breastfed children"* (Alex). These findings concur with themes 1, 2, 3 and 5, 6 in Beck and Watson's (2008) study examining the impact of birth trauma on breastfeeding. However, they differ in that none of the women felt their body was violated by breastfeeding which was a theme in the Beck and Watson (2008) study. Future pregnancies and births were another potentially redemptive opportunity. The desire to complete their family overrode their heartfelt fear of childbirth. All women reported an assumption that the worst had already happened and their second birth had to be better. They held on to this belief in order to override their fear. This assumption was not identified in the Thomson and Downe (2010) study which examined women's experience of a positive birth after a traumatic one. However, there is concurrence in the preparation the women undertook in order to give themselves the best chance of the birth they desired. They were determined to listen to their own bodies and act upon it, not be dominated by experts, to ask for help, to build relationships with appropriate staff, and in the case of Joanne to read her medical notes. Only Sandy achieved that redemptive birth and the vindication, satisfaction and confidence that it brought and which has been noted in the Thomson and Downe (2010) study. Sadly for Joanne and Diane, difficult second births brought their childbearing years to a premature end, as the fear and risk of future births was too large to bear. For Alex, the powerful combination of her body's failure and of a world over which she had no control for a third time, was horrifying, resulting in grieving and three months of *"hell"* as she sank into depression (Alex).

Traumatic birth had an impact on marital relationships, and in this study the women focused on support, or lack of it. Two women, Sandy and Diane, felt completely let down by their partners during the birth. They had silently cried for help and protection and they had felt it unforthcoming. Even whilst acknowledging that their husbands could not be expected to know what to do, the women felt terribly angry and resentful. This anger seemed to spill into the early days of motherhood when they shut their partners out, focused on their baby, and felt unable to give consideration to their partner's feelings. Other studies have also found disruption to the relationship due to lack of partner empathy (Allen 1998; Ayers et al. 2006). The other two women reported on the support from their partners in the aftermath of the trauma, which ultimately brought them closer together as a couple. Whilst a common theme in other studies has been the negative impact on couples' sex lives (Allen 1998; Nichols and

Ayers 2007), this was only mentioned by one participant who reported that sex became more painful. Previous studies have found problems in mother–baby bonding (Reynolds 1997; Ballard et al. 1995; Ayers et al. 2006). This research concurred as two women spoke of initial bonding issues. Whilst this is not uncommon in the general population, the nature of the trauma seems to be the causation. Reid (2011) has noted that some mothers have difficulty separating the trauma from their baby. This appears to be the case with Joanne who attributed her initial bonding problems to her physical injuries caused by the birth (Joanne). Sadly, her child now experiences guilt that her birth caused her mother's condition. This has caused Joanne further regret and guilt. Alex's serious medical condition occurred after the birth and the baby was an adverse strength-sapping responsibility (Alex). Alex later compensated for her initial feelings with hyper-vigilant, overprotective behaviour, *"I wouldn't let her out of my sight"*. Sandy's attachment behaviour whilst similar was all encompassing from the very start as she immediately fell in love with her baby. These attachment patterns have also been found in other studies (e.g. Allen 1998; Ayers et al. 2006; Nichols and Ayers 2007).

Post-traumatic growth was attributed to their trauma. The growth was identified in terms of increased personal strength, relating to others and new possibilities. There was a collective feeling that if *"you can get through this you can get through anything"* (Joanne). The trauma and its consequences had forced them to look at, get to know and question themselves and their assumptive worlds. Diane said this process *"helped me develop as a person"*. Their trauma left them wanting to, and knowing that they could, help others. For some, there was a direct correlation between their trauma and wanting to become a Counsellor. Unfortunately, there appears to be a paucity of research on birth trauma and PTG with which to compare findings. However, a study by Souza et al. (2009) found an existential element to growth in a group of Brazilian women who had suffered a near death experience in childbirth. This is in contrast to this study where no one reported a new appreciation of life or spiritual growth. There may be two reasons for this. Firstly, the birth traumas were of a different nature, with one group of women aware that they had been close to death; none of the participants of this study said they thought they might die, although they were frightened. It would make sense that a near death experience would make life more precious. And perhaps Brazil is arguably a more religious society than the UK, which may explain the spiritual growth. However the timing of the Souza study is also problematic, as participants were interviewed within six weeks of their birth trauma, arguably too early to label this as PTG (Calhoun and Tedeschi, 1998) and too early to know whether this 'growth' was sustainable. The existence of PTG did not mean their trauma was forgotten, forgiven or healed. There was a duality to their experiences. Growth was not the only long-term consequence. Between them, the women were also left with regret, guilt, and some fragility.

Research suggests that as many as one in three women would describe their birth experience as traumatic and as a consequence have experienced post-traumatic stress symptoms (Creedy et al. 2000; Soet et al. 2003; Ayers et al. 2009). However the focus of post-natal care is with the physical rather than psychological (Peeler et al. 2013) and for a number of reasons, many women will move out of the post-natal care system without receiving any psychological help. Whilst most hospitals offer some form of post-natal service, the offering differs from hospital to hospital (Peeler et al. 2013), with most of the services (78%) being a medical debriefing rather than a psychological debriefing (Ayers et al. 2007). This debriefing usually involves just one session, with the mother going through her notes with medical staff in order to gain a better understanding of the birth. One might even question whether there is the potential that one session may indeed increase distress rather than decrease it (Ayers et al. 2007).

Given the magnitude of the problem, it is probable that an individual Counsellor will work with clients who have endured a traumatic birth. This research has highlighted some important challenges and implications for counselling practice. All the participants in this research had previously displayed a reluctance to talk about their experience and their feelings. Indeed, despite the elapsed time, the self-development involved in their Counsellor training and personal therapy, it was the first time any participant had talked about the trauma and impact in any detail. A complex web of feelings including failure, inadequacy, disappoint-ment, loss and a fear of making it real created a silence that was hard to break. And these feelings may also have concerned others who were most dear to the participants. Consider the difficulty in expressing the guilt, shame and sorrow surrounding bonding problems, how disloyal and frighten-ing it might be to express feelings of anger towards and being let down by your partner; how vulnerable a woman might feel to describe giving birth, a natural process, as traumatic. Any Counsellor would do well to reflect on Rogers' six necessary and sufficient conditions to therapeutic growth (1957). Regardless of the individual Counsellor's therapeutic framework, surely the safety and space to explore such sensitive emotions will be dependent on the Counsellor's ability to offer empathy, respect and congruence. Given that PND and PTSD have some commonalities there is the risk that some women will be misdiagnosed with PND, the more familiar condition, when PTSD may be more appropriate (White et al. 2006). Counsellors may therefore find themselves working with misdiagnosed clients and they should be aware of this possibility. It is important that Counsellors are sensitive to what Joseph and Linley (2008) call 'red flag behaviours', are aware of their own level of competency and do not walk blindly into an area of suffering which might cause further harm to a client.

Conclusion

There are limitations to this research which is general to all phenomenological studies. It is a small-scale study, of self-defined experiences from women from a similar geographical area. Malim et al. (1992) argue IPA studies have the potential to be subjective, intuitive and impressionistic. IPA recognizes that understanding requires interpretation which could mean that another researcher would interpret the data differently. And whilst reflexivity will moderate interpretation, it would be impossible to remove it completely. Some will still view these points as researcher bias (Willig 2008). Denzin and Lincoln (2005) highlight that the success of interviews is dependent on the participant's ability to report on their experience. And there will always be questions about the reliability of using participant's retrospective recollections. Furthermore, Parahoo (1997) regards volunteer sampling as weak, as participants are motivated to volunteer for some reason and this should be acknowledged as a potential sampling bias. In order to ensure ethical practice, participants were qualified Counsellors whose training necessitates personal development. They may have worked through their traumatic birth and be in a very different place to women who have never had the opportunity to explore their experience. Participants were also at least fifteen years post-trauma and again could be in a different place from mothers who have experienced the trauma more recently.

However, phenomenologically this does not invalidate its meaning. The interview process produced rich information. But after the initial analysis it would have been beneficial to return to the participants for further illumination. The aim of this phenomenological study was to gain a rich in-depth understanding of the impact of traumatic childbirth. The research questions focused on how participants processed their experience and how it impacted on their lives. Participants reported feelings of anger, fear, shock and being out of control during their birth. They were initially left with a sense of failure, inadequacy and weakness. The birth trauma impacted on marital relationships, the mother and baby bond and attachment behaviour. It was also a major consideration in decisions about future pregnancies, bringing childbearing to a premature end for half of the participants.

The research showed that the participants employed a number of coping mechanisms in order to protect themselves from the horror of the reality. Dissociation and repression were common features in the aftermath of the trauma. Focusing on their healthy baby allowed the mothers to stay in the present and limit rumination. None of the women had been diagnosed with, nor tested for PTSD. However, all the women stated they suffered from depression in the aftermath of the trauma. As there are commonalities in the symptoms of PTSS and depression, the possibility that some of the participants had PTSS should not be ruled out. The women worked through their depression in different ways but the importance of support was noted. Finally, PTG in terms of increased personal strength, relating to others and new possibilities were attributed to the trauma and the aftermath. However, this growth exists alongside other less desirable outcomes such as regret, guilt and fragility. Traumatic childbirth, feelings of failure, guilt, bonding issues, relationship issues, and the physical repercussions are all difficult things to admit and talk about. This is made harder by society's rose-tinted view of motherhood, and the perception that the end justifies the means. The fact that the participants had never spoken in any depth about their birth trauma, despite the considerable time lapse, is testament to this difficulty. It is evident that, even today, there is no standard offering of postpartum psychological care for women who have suffered a birth trauma (Peeler et al. 2013). Given the potential scale of this issue, the impact on the individual and the potential repercussions on the family and therefore society at large, it would seem sensible to devote resource to this area of research, in particular the type of support which would be beneficial. It would also seem appropriate to offer screening and monitoring of postpartum women in order to be able to offer suitable support at the appropriate time.

CHAPTER SIX

THE EXPERIENCES OF PERSON-CENTRED COUNSELLORS WHO WORK WITH CLIENTS WHO PRESENT WITH COMPLICATED GRIEF

Eleanor Warman

Introduction

This chapter focuses on the experiences of Person-Centred Counsellors who have worked with clients who present with Complicated Grief (CG). Loss and grief are universal (Howarth 2011). If grief is the price we pay for love (Parkes and Prigerson 2010), then most humans, essentially relational creatures (Mearns and Thorne 2013), will experience forms of loss and grief. While most bereavements, though painful, progress without issue, between 4% (Marwit 1996) and 40% (Newson et al. 2011) of grievers suffer complications. If we do not live in a vacuum, neither do we grieve in one (Humphrey 2009). Cultural norms and expectations vary along with individuals (Cutcliffe 1998). Changing demographics and family structures combine with complex modern societal requirements to contribute to inherent difficulties in the grieving process (Gaudio 1998). Additionally, with bereavement increasingly medicalized and the wider secularization of society, people are turning to GPs, or Counsellors, for support (Payne et al. 2002). This upturn in demand for bereavement counselling raises a question concerning the position and healing potential offered by the Person-Centred Approach (PCA) in relation to grief. It could be suggested the PCA stands on the fringes of grief theory, with loss and grief 'a greatly neglected area in Person-Centred literature' (Bryant-Jefferies 2006, p. viii). However, with grief so unique, and clients sensitive to societal expectations, there seems to me to be a close fit between the therapeutic needs of bereaved clients and the ethos of the PCA, though the tension between this phenomenologically based support and more externally structured dictates of a CG diagnosis may prove problematic.

My interest in CG stems from working as a Counsellor in a hospice, and my work with the charity Cruse. I have no significant personal experience of bereavement through death. This led me to familiarize myself with CG as a diagnosable condition. While every client I have seen shares hallmarks in their grief, the uniqueness of their experience is undeniable. The extremity of some grief reactions has proved challenging, and one client in particular could be deemed to be experiencing CG, though I was not aware of this term during our work. Societal expectations about grief have proved problematic for every client to some extent, high-lighting the need for a neutral space, such as counselling, in which to explore their own reactions safely. However, this need highlights the impact of such work on those who undertake it, leading to my interest in how it is to work with bereaved clients experiencing such reactions, and what is needed by the Counsellor to sustain such work. I am interested in the implications of working in this way; the deep roots and extremes of CG pose a potential challenge for all Counsellors, but perhaps especially for Person-Centred Counsellors, whose adherence to the core conditions means tracking the client closely, and entering their frame of reference.

The main aim of my study is to explore how Person-Centred Counsellors make sense of their work with clients who they deem to be experiencing CG. Within this, I seek to explore personal challenges and experiences, and self-care issues along with issues around the central theoretical tenets such as congruence, empathy and unconditional positive regard. CG had been proposed for inclusion in DSM-V, but ultimately this did not happen, although Persistent Complex Bereavement Disorder, a seemingly equivalent condition, does appear in a secondary rubric. However, the abundance of writing on the subject and multiplicity of viewpoints brought grief, and its presentations, into sharp focus within the counselling practice community. While I in no way intend my findings to be prescriptive, I feel this research still serves as a useful and informative source for those interested in working with the bereaved, as well as opening up opportunities for further research. My research question is: What are the experiences of Person-Centred Counsellors who have worked with clients who present with Complicated Grief?

What the literature says

Loss and grief are universal (Howarth 2011), but the ways we grieve are wide-ranging. My research does not focus on grief theory, per se, but for context I offer a brief overview. Freud (1917) asserted the key to successful mourning was severing emotional attachment with the deceased; the 'work of mourning'. Ideas of mourning as something one 'does', remained prominent in theory for decades (Stroebe and Schut 1999). Bowlby (1980) suggested three phases of grief, later increased to four (numbing, yearning/searching, disorganization/despair and reorganization) through which grievers oscillate. Parkes proposed phases of grief: disbelief, yearning, anger, depression and acceptance (Parkes and Prigerson 2010). According to Silverman and Klass (1996), Parkes' path to resolution came from severing attachment, rather than maintaining continued bonds with the deceased. Kubler-Ross' (1969) five stages of grief (denial, anger, bargaining, depression and acceptance) originated from research with the dying. They, and other stage theories, have been widely adopted as illustrative of an expected journey for the bereaved (Wortman and Cohen Silver 1989; Littlewood 1992; Bonanno 2009; Worden 2010). However, following stage theories literally can result in grievers' natural oscillations being overlooked or deemed abnormal (Wortman and Cohen Silver 1989; Sprang and McNeil 1995; Bonanno 2009). Worden (2010) proposed a task-based theory. These tasks, which Worden explains do not have a required order, aim to give mourners some sense that action can be taken in adjusting. Tasks consist of accepting the reality of the loss, processing the pain of grief, adjusting to a world without the deceased, and finding a way to retain connection whilst embarking on a new life. Rando (2013) suggested six Rs; recognize the loss, react to the separation, recollect the deceased, relinquish old attachments, readjust and reinvest. These processes are set within three phases of mourning (avoidance, confrontation, accommodation). The final processes (i.e. readjust and reinvest) offer a bridge between classic theories (severing emotional attachment) and newer ideas (retaining bonds while moving forward) (Litsa 2013). Silverman and Klass (1996) describe continuing bonds, while the Dual Process Model proposed by Stroebe and Schut (1999) offers a model in which the fluid nature of grief (Haugh 2012) is taken into account, with regular oscillation between loss-oriented coping and restoration-oriented coping patterns. Whether viewed from a stage, task or phase-based viewpoint, negotiating loss is painful (Haugh 2012). Most grievers experience symptoms to a degree, but return to pre-loss functioning relatively soon (Bonanno et al. 2007). For some, however, the path of grief becomes too much to traverse, and complications arise.

While there are strong calls not to pathologize grief (e.g. Shear et al. 2001; Love 2007; Simon 2012; Fox and Jones 2013), studies have identified that in some cases, grieving goes awry. Figures on grievers suffering complications have numbers ranging between 4% and 20% of cases resulting in a complication (Marwit 1996; Golden and Dalgleish 2012), with Newson et al. (2011) suggesting that as high as 40% of grievers are at risk of CG. There is no official CG definition, but proposed inclusion as a new disorder for the DSM-V meant much attention was paid to consolidating data and opinion over recent years. This resulted in criteria which seem broadly accepted as signifiers of a CG reaction. 'Persistent yearning' for the deceased is a major criterion, universally agreed upon (Gort 1984; Kyriakopoulos 2008). 'Intrusive thoughts or images' are cited by many as another criterion (Prigerson et al. 1996; Shear 2012). 'Prolonged anger or bitterness' features prominently in the criteria (Jeffreys 2005; Prigerson and Maciejewski 2006) as do 'denial of the reality of' the death (Jacobs and Prigerson 2000; Harvard Medical School 2006) and 'increased social isolation' (Shear et al. 2001; MacCallum and Bryant 2011). 'Increased suicidality' is the next criterion to be widely supported (Latham and Prigerson 2004; Simon 2012) followed by a 'sense of purposelessness' (Howarth 2011; Shear 2012) and 'intense loneliness or emotion' (Jacobs and Prigerson 2000; Simon 2012). Criteria that are less commonly referenced, are 'extreme avoidance' of reminders of the deceased (Shear and Mulhare 2008; Howarth 2011) and 'physical manifestations' (Gort 1984; Simon 2012). The inability to return to 'normal' life after the death is a key factor in deeming a grief reaction complicated (Bonanno 2009; Simon 2012). Similarly, while many symptoms ascribed to CG are reminiscent of normal acute grief reactions, in CG, they remain fresh and intense for at least six months minimum post-bereavement (Shear et al. 2001; Prigerson 2004). It is this duration and intensity which signifies deviation from the norm (Shear and Mulhare 2008; Howarth 2011; Shear 2012). As well as symptomatic similarities to acute grief, CG also shares traits of disorders including major depression and PTSD (Harvard Medical School 2006; Machin 2009). While symptomatic similarities are evident, symptom clusters are argued to be distinct from those of depression or anxiety (Prigerson 2004; Boelen et al. 2010). Studies have shown that treating CG equivalently to PTSD, or depression, is ineffective in reducing CG symptoms (e.g. Shear and Mulhare 2008). Therefore, recognizing CG as a valid disorder allows targeted treatment, and crucially to the American context, creates options for treating CG via health insurance. However, the idea of an official diagnosable condition is met with resistance. The uniqueness of grief is emphasized throughout the literature (Cutcliffe 1998; Rubin et al. 2012) and there are fears that a CG label risks pathologizing or medicalizing grief (Love 2007; Fox and Jones 2013). The emerging complexity of interconnecting elements influencing grief leads Machin (2009) to posit that a definition of CG is, as a result, elusive. Critics also suggest that diagnostic categorization of 'normal' comes from a solidly Western viewpoint (Rosenblatt 2013), potentially ignoring global cultural subtleties in grieving patterns. However, the criterion proposed by Shear (2012) does include cultural consideration with regards to time span. CG, itself, seems to be an umbrella term under which other grief reactions are placed. CG is often used interchangeably with Prolonged Grief Disorder (PGD) (Boelen and van den Bout 2008; Wittouck et al. 2011) but, for many, PGD is widely regarded as simply one form of CG (Rando, et al. 2012; Rando 2013). Worden (2010) offers his paradigm for complicated mourning in the form of four headings (delayed, chronic, exaggerated and masked grief reactions), with symptoms echoing those discussed above. Bowlby (1980) spoke of 'mislocating' the deceased, positing chronic mourning and prolonged absence of grieving as examples of pathological grief, while Parkes and Prigerson (2010) offer PGD and delayed grief as complications. Others, too, use CG as an umbrella, with different labels for CG reactions including chronic grief, pathological grief, abnormal grief, traumatic grief, absent or distorted grief, delayed grief, identification or mummification (Littlewood 1992). CG research shows there are factors which influence the likelihood of developing a CG reaction. These include the nature of the loss, nature of the attachment, previous losses, culture and the griever's personality or world view (Field and Filanosky 2010; Mancini et al. 2011) as well as age (Newson et al. 2011), and cognitive functioning (MacCallum and Bryant 2011). This adds weight to grief as a unique experience, but because my research focuses on the experiences of Counsellors rather than clients, I shall not visit these factors in more detail.

With grief theory changing, and society's expectations of grievers often at odds with their own feelings (McLaren 1998), Bereavement Counsellors' willingness to allow exploration of unique grief reactions appears much needed. Consequently, there is a need for exploration of the nature of the role, and its impact on those who undertake it. In 1998 Kirchberg et al. suggested there was 'little empirical research on the reactions of therapists and counselors' working with issues of around death, 'despite growing concern' with vicarious traumatization (p. 100). In subsequent years, studies have emerged which begin a picture of the challenges and joys of being a Bereavement Counsellor. A basic challenge that emerges is the likelihood that bereavement work will trigger anxieties about the Counsellor's own losses (Lamb 1988), as well as feared losses (Barlow and Phelan 2007; Worden 2010). This links with increased death awareness, and existential anxieties around living day-to-day with the vulnerable nature of life (Kirchberg et al. 1998; Becvar 2003; Dunphy and Schniering 2009; Worden 2010). The ability to sit comfortably with high, intense emotions may apply to all Counsellor roles, but is singled out as a quality necessary for Bereavement Counsellors (Gaudio 1998; Puterbaugh 2008; Worden 2010). Studies suggest Bereavement Counsellors can struggle with feelings of frustration or anger (e.g. Worden 2010). This stems from the way grief is experienced by clients, making it hard for Bereavement Counsellors to feel of significant use (Lamb 1988; Kirchberget al. 1998; Worden 2010). Bowlby (1980) spoke of feeling impotent in the face of client pain, while McLaren (1998) referred to 'the invisible therapist syndrome'. Working constantly in the face of such emotions can leave Bereavement Counsellors vulnerable to vicarious traumatization (Kirchberg et al. 1998) or compassion fatigue (Becvar 2003). This work may carry the greatest risk for Counsellors who are inexperienced in the field. Specifically, novice Counsellors can find topics around death and loss to be anxiety-provoking, more than their experienced colleagues (Kirchberg et al. 1998). Even experienced Counsellors with little background of relevant training, or client contact, can experience discomfort around death and grief (Kirchberg et al. 1998). Ensuring that the Counsellors' own losses are adequately dealt with is regarded as vital preparation for dealing with loss and grief work (Gaudio 1998; Puterbaugh 2008; Humphrey 2009; Worden 2010). Vital, perhaps, because the aforementioned anxiety-provoking reaction was found to be especially pronounced for Counsellors with pre-existing death fear (Kirchberg et al. 1998). Bereavement counselling can be a strain on Counsellors' emotional and spiritual resources (Becvar 2003). It is proposed that Counsellors, working with grief and loss, also experience intense emotional and mental states (Dunphy and Schniering 2009) in a wraparound experience, touching them emotionally, mentally, physically and spiritually (Puterbaugh 2008). It is therefore deemed essential that Bereavement Counsellors be open and knowledgeable about their internal dialogues and feelings (Gaudio 1998; Browning 2003) and be ready to acknowledge and act upon limitations and vulnerabilities (Becvar 2003; Worden 2010). Personal maturity, deep sense of perspective and acceptance of death are proposed by Josef as necessary attributes of Bereavement Counsellors (cited in Dunphy and Schniering 2009). A holistic approach to self-care is encouraged (Becvar 2003; Puterbaugh 2008; Humphrey 2009), with time spent with like-minded professionals deemed a vital component (Becvar 2003; Wheeler-Roy and Amyot 2004; Puterbaugh 2008). It seems, therefore, that the lived-experience of Bereavement Counsellors is critical to their work (Dunphy and Schniering 2009). Bereavement counselling is shown to bring joys as well as challenges. The work is described as being satisfying (Becvar 2003; Puterbaugh 2008), with much gained for the Counsellor from acting as witness to the client's spirit and struggle; McLaren (1998) speaks of feeling enriched, Becvar (2003) enjoys enhancement in treasuring the mundane as well as the magnificent, while Browning (2003) calls the work exhilarating, and Puterbaugh (2008) references the spiritual aspects of the work.

Many assert that the individuality of clients' grief be recognized and respected (e.g. Wortman and Cohen Silver

1989; Jones 1995; Sprang and McNeil 1995; McLaren 1998; Muller and Thompson 2003; Servaty-Seib 2004; Humphrey 2009; Haugh 2012; Rubin et al. 2012). Therefore, the client-led ethos of Person-Centred Counselling, with its non-judgemental prizing of the client (Rogers 1979), where the individual's experience is heard and accepted (Haugh 2012), would seem to complement that assertion. However, the paucity of findings from my search leads me to conclude that the Person-Centred Approach has historically lacked any serious voice in the theory of grief and bereavement counselling. The majority of grief literature stems from a psychodynamic perspective (McLaren 1998), where the belief in finite amounts of available energy shines a logical light on the idea of tasks or stages, and a working towards 'letting go' (Haugh 2012) as in the work of Freud, Bowlby, Worden and Kubler-Ross. Searches turned up few results which could be deemed Person-Centred. Haugh (2012) wrote a comprehensive chapter on a Person-Centred theoretical approach to loss and bereavement, while Bryant-Jefferies' (2006) book takes the form of dramatized accounts of counselling and supervision sessions focused on death from the viewpoint of a Person-Centred Counsellor. These Person-Centred bereavement works are complemented by an article by Jan McLaren (1998), detailing her experiences as a Person-Centred Bereavement Counsellor. The individuality of a client's grief seems to me to fit with the PCA. Browning (2003) suggests authentic engagement with a client is facilitated by a level of informed not-knowing, with client, rather than Counsellor, regarded as expert on their experiences; this resonates with Mearns and Thorne (2013) in their assertion that the mantle of expert is to be avoided by Person-Centred Counsellors. Servaty-Seib (2004) also suggests the emphasis on individual phenomenological experience makes the

Person-Centred framework appropriate for bereaved clients, while Bryant-Jefferies (2006) describes honouring the uniqueness of each client's path, rather than suggesting passing through stages, which have been criticized for not addressing individual idiosyncrasies (Sprang and McNeil 1995). Haugh (2012), however, suggests stage theories can help the Counsellor stay in the room, and accept what they see and hear without feeling overwhelmed by what they witness. Machin (2009) considers that Person-Centred Counsellors must be able to distinguish between unacceptable actions which may present themselves in times of high grief, and the innate worth of the client and, further, places emphasize on how attention to the core conditions and Counsellor's self allows this. Attention to the client's frame of reference allows the Counsellor to explore how the client's self-created 'microcosmic social world' and their idea of the 'me' is affected by the loss of the significant other who has been written into this world (Littlewood 1992, p. 72). This attention to the client's inner world may be especially helpful for those who feel that their grief does not fit others' expectations of normal, possibly because modern society shies away from public expressions of grief (Gort 1984; Parkes and Prigerson 2010) despite grief being widely regarded as a social process (Littlewood 1992). Person-Centred theory can help explain why clients experience different reactions (Haugh 2012). Archer (1999) suggests it is the alteration in self-concept which accompanies external changes, such as bereavement, which is regarded as being crucial for the resolution of grief. Servaty-Seib (2004) gives a detailed view of how Person-Centred theory fits with bereavement: grieving can become difficult when obstacles such as conditions of worth, and their subsequent prescription for how to mourn, are placed in the client's way. This attention to an external locus of evaluation often leads to disparity between self-concept and the client's genuine experience. Thus Person-Centred Counselling offers a critical opportunity for clients to regain a subjective sense of their own individual experiencing. Bryant-Jefferies (2006) agrees that clients' bereavement experience tends to be affected by the conditioning effects of their past experiences. There are drawbacks, or limitations, to the idea of Person-Centred bereavement counselling. Bereaved clients, especially those deemed as experiencing CG, suffer feelings of isolation and confusion, have difficulty sleeping and feel numb or removed from life. In the face of the resultant potential difficulty engaging, this may impact the relationship in terms of Rogers' first necessary and sufficient condition, that two people must be in psychological contact (1957). For the relationship to work the client must be able to engage to an extent, which may not always be possible with bereaved clients. Bereavement Counsellors can be said to travel the journey of loss alongside the client (Machin 2009), but a client's expression of grief may be just the start, with the PCA criticized for lacking focus on mourning and coping, once the expression of grief has been achieved (Servaty-Seib 2004). If more complex Counsellor-led interactions are indeed deemed necessary, this may sit in tension with the non-directive client-led basis of Person-Centred Counselling. One example of this may be the normalization of grief reactions. Many clients are overwhelmed by the breadth and strength of their reactions. Especially keen are fears that they are going mad, or in my own counselling experience, that they are a terrible person for their vehement reactions to seeing 'in-tact' units, i.e. couples or families. In advising, or even suggesting, to clients that their reactions are 'normal', McLaren (1998) posits that the Counsellor deviates from Person-Centred practice and assumes an authority role, disempowering the client. She then states, however, that she believes normalization aids the empathic relationship, allowing the client to feel understood, less isolated and thus better able to understand, and accept, their own reactions (1998). Haugh (2012), while finding empathic reaction usually sufficient, does concede that on occasion failure to respond to questions of normality from clients is tantamount to avoidance, and therefore incongruence on the Person-Centred Counsellor's part.

Participants

Purposive sampling was chosen. Criteria for recruitment were specific, ensuring my sampling avoided being deemed haphazard (Flick 2011). These included:

- Trained Person-Centred Counsellors, qualified to at least diploma level.
- At least two years post qualification.
- Able to discuss in depth at least one example of working in a Person-Centred way with a client presenting with complicated grief, within the last five years.
- Currently in practice as Counsellor or supervisor.
- Currently in supervision.
- Access to personal counselling if required.
- Member of BACP or equivalent professional organization.

The criterion for participant exclusion was: Counsellors who are known to me personally (from practice, university, personal counselling or supervision). Recruitment began with an advert on Therapytoday.net on the BACP Research noticeboard, and with requests for adverts to be placed in selected hospices and counselling practices around the North

West. Two participants came from one hospice, the third following a suggestion from my practice co-ordinator, and the fourth came following a suggestion by an existing participant. The participants were all white Europeans, three women and one man, with a range of between five and twenty years' experience in a bereavement setting, and varied experience of other practices outside bereavement.

Data collection

Data collection was via audio-recorded, semi-structured interviews. I designed the interview structure to consist of eight open questions with prompts:

- Your previous experience working with bereaved clients.
- Brief outline of the client you would like to discuss, their presentation, why you chose to bring them today.
- Your feelings working with this client, both during your work, after the work ended and now.
- Any challenges working with this client.
- Your process around the core conditions and frame of reference when working with this client.
- The role of supervision in your work with this client.
- Discussion of any other clients presenting with complicated grief who impacted upon you or brought up issues which feel relevant to this and you would like to discuss.
- Anything else you would like to say.

Participants were interviewed in a suitable location of their choice, in the order in which they became available.

Findings

A thematic analysis revealed three master themes, divided into thirteen sub-themes. Within that, two sub-themes are broken into further topics where the data offered 'snapshots' of valuable insight, and the smaller topics fitted together coherently.

1 – Shifting Sands: Movement Moment and Malleability in the Counselling Room	2 – The Self of the Counsellor	3 – Role of and within the Therapeutic Relationship

1.1 Working on different levels
1.2 Tangible vs intangible
1.3 Ideas of movement
1.4 Chronology; time is not linear
	2.1 Impact on self: positive
	2.2 Impact on self: negative
	2.3 Self-care;
	   2.3.1 General
	   2.3.2 Supervision
	   2.3.3 Team
	2.4 Counsellor as tool; narrative reflecting process
		3.1 Counsellor as witness
		3.2 The experience of experience
		3.3 Relationship as 'our' tool
		3.4 Views on the role;
		   3.4.1 Suicide
		   3.4.2 Nature of bereavement
		   3.4.3 Labels
		   3.4.4 'It's what I'm there for'

Table 10. Master, sub-themes and sub-sub-themes.

Master theme 1: Shifting Sands; Movement, Moment and Malleability in the Counselling Room.

A prominent feature of my findings was the idea that much of the counselling process, as experienced by participants, feels ephemeral or unfixed. I had a sense of emerging malleability as I undertook each analysis, and this was borne out in the subsequent emergent themes and this overarching master theme.

Sub-theme 1.1: Working on different levels: The notion of simultaneous experiences in the counselling room seemed strong. Sometimes personal feelings operated on different levels: *"It felt sad but happy* [when we ended]*"* (Lisa). Sometimes it was participants' professional selves displaying dual levels of operation: *"There was an aspect of me* [normalizing physical symptoms] *and another part of me thinking 'my God is he going to have a heart attack?'"*. (Dawn). *"It's balancing on that holding in mind the freedom of any person, and the need for care in any person"* (Marie). *"She doesn't present in any way that makes me feel I have to be concerned about it, but it's something that's there in my mind"* (Stephen). *"It's just staying with that feeling with it and but also using it"* (Lisa). This duality extends to tensions between Counsellor and organizational preferences: [Ending with the client felt OK on a personal level but] *"maybe it felt also ok, I don't have to justify* [number of sessions to management]*"* (Dawn).

Sub-theme 1.2: Tangible vs intangible: Tangible and intangible layers of process seem to be experienced by participants: *"*[Suicide is] *also tangible in so far that she's not really rooted here anymore"* (Marie). This may hold a literal 'tangible' element, referenced by Marie, while also offering intangibility in the fact the client is rootless and drifting. It also feels suicide in itself is hard to grasp, contributing to the layered nuances of this statement. Marie makes another striking statement: *"Because of the gap that doesn't seem to be there for* [the client]*"* (Marie). The issue for her client is that the gap in timeframe from childhood to adulthood does not exist. Similarly, a gap itself does not 'exist', it is an intangible space. In not existing, the gap seems to change form into something more tangible that can be identified and verbalized. Stephen experienced moments of (in)tangibility, where awareness is concrete but the more tangible workings cannot be pinned down: *"I don't know exactly how that works, but I'm very aware of that"* (Stephen). Dawn too witnessed tangible moments with clients. *"It would be quite painful to be in a room with him because it was palpable how much he was hurting … It was kind of like electric in the room when he was telling me about that … She wanted to wear* [her grief]" (Dawn).

Sub-theme 1.3: Ideas of movement: Senses of movement were depicted through metaphorical representation by participants. The differing qualities of movement were striking; while reference is made to *"walking with"* clients (Marie) and that *"people generally do move forward"* (Lisa), not uncommon in reference to the counselling journey. Other images offer a less controlled process: *"With her it's like on the on the edge of life and death (teetering)"* (Marie); *"She brings me in all sorts of kind of waters (rapids)"* (Marie); *"It was sort of spilling out … into the rest of my life"* (Stephen); *"The feelings started to flood in"* (Lisa); *"[Emotions] swinging from being very, very sad to very angry"* (Lisa); and *"Felt a bit like launching, ready to launch into life again"* (Lisa).

Sub-theme 1.4: Chronology; time is not linear: The final sub-theme of master theme 1 deals with participants' experience of time. I felt that within the counselling relationship, ideas of time as a linear concept did not always apply, for both Counsellor and client. Marie speaks of her client's fractured timeline; one illustrative example was the idea of the possible 'end' being present from the start of the relationship: *"Bang in the middle* [of their decision to work together] *do I continue living?"* (Marie). Participants speak of their clients' past being very present: *"Being with her, erm, as an abused child"* (Marie); *"She talks as if … it is happening now"* (Marie); *"[This incident] took her back into* [her childhood abuse]" (Stephen); *"[His connection to the deceased was] very current, absolutely current … He felt safest at home because that's where she was"* (Dawn). For some it is their own feelings which remain current: *"And that really got me, yeah. It does get to me,* *that"* (Stephen); *"I was just so moved by that, still am, it was a few years ago and still am"* (Dawn).

Master theme 2 – The Self of the Counsellor.

Counselling work may impact the Counsellor, with participants reporting that the work was both beneficial and also potentially damaging or difficult. Within this master theme, I divided the sub-theme of self-care into General, Supervision and Team, because I felt the participants' views on supervision and team to be worth reflecting.

Sub-theme: 2.1: Impact on self: positive: Personal emotional fulfilment seemed a common benefit: *"I find counselling in itself such a rewarding role"* (Marie). *"Also very inspiring I think"* (Dawn). *"It's beautiful work, really, moving work. It's a privilege to be with people"* (Dawn). *"It's rewarding and I get a lot of satisfaction out of it"* (Lisa). Intellectual fulfilment also seemed rewarded: *"Being witness to people's process, I think it's incredibly intriguing ... that interaction between theory and practice, theory, practice, forever ... I think is, is there a better job? I don't think so"* (Marie). *"For me to hear people chewing over what's going on for them, I just find the most fascinating thing in life"* (Stephen). *"He taught me stuff as well"* (Lisa). For Lisa, preparation for the future benefited from work with clients: *"Positive feelings about myself really as a person, and also in terms of preparing for ultimately sadnesses in my own life"* (Lisa). While for Dawn, spiritual benefits were an important aspect of her work: *"Given that I have certain spiritual beliefs for me that was kind of very affirming ... It's the opportunity for the spiritual"* (Dawn).

Sub-theme 2.2: Impact on self: negative: However, it is perhaps unsurprising that working with such pain and emotion can leave participants vulnerable to negative impact. Feelings of incompetence, or doubt, were common to all participants. Sometimes the impact seems physical. In discussing not wanting to pressurize a suicidal client by phoning too soon, yet wanting her to know she cares, Marie seemed weighed down by this delicate balance. Other participants expressed physical impact: *"You know, that real kind of* [squeals twice] *can't do this can't do this"* (Dawn). *"I did feel very drained, and feel like I need to go* [exhales] *you know, kind of just shake it all out"* (Lisa). Three of the four participants referred to clients somatizing symptoms. Two participants referenced this as being a challenge. While sometimes, there seemed a sense of impending danger of a more emotional sense: *"The challenge is really in sticking with it and standing near to the fire'* (Marie)". *"At the moment my head's a bit burnt out with it … To actually deeply empathise with that I think is one of the … most likely aspects of vicarious traumatisation for me"* (Stephen). *"I was completely oblivious to the cost, to me of working in that environment"* (Dawn).

Sub-theme 2.3: Self-care: Given the potential for harm to Counsellor and client in this work, I found self-care to be a strong theme for the participants. Supervision and the impact of a team have been presented as distinguishable topics within this self-care sub-theme.

Sub-sub-theme 2.3.1): General: Participants' feelings around self-care seem to reject the idea it is *"a package or … a pill you take"* (Marie), and instead, the feeling is more of a wider-lived experience. *"It's a way of living … I wonder whether it's become second nature to have that monitoring of … well-being, balance"* (Marie). *"For me it's about being my all, but it means about me having spaces to recuperate"* (Stephen). *"I didn't balance my life there enough with life-affirming activities, and I think if you're going to work around bereavement and death* [you must]*"* (Dawn). *"I've done this job for a long time and … I just have ways of coping and … good friendships and I make sure that I have a good fun time outside of work"* (Lisa). There seems almost an element of surrendering involved: *"With clients who are kind of verging in that direction, it seems to me it's more a spiritual kind of type of support and searching … it's kind of a surrender to a general system of care for something that is less tangible"* (Marie). *"There's something about just accepting life and death as it is really"* (Lisa).

Sub-sub-theme 2.3.2: Supervision: Specific references to supervision indicate it is an important element of Counsellor self-care.

Sub-sub-theme 2.3.3: Team: However, the *"gift of working in a team"* (Marie) also seemed intrinsic to Counsellor self-care. *"Being part of a very good team is probably my main support in my work"* (Marie). *"To have an immediate, supportive er bunch of you know professionals around me, both within and around counselling, works really well for me"* (Stephen).

Sub theme 2.3.4: Counsellor as tool: narrative reflecting process: The final sub-theme is included under 'self'; it seemed that verbal reflection of any process can only come from the *self* of the person who speaks it. At times, the narrative style of participants seemed to reflect the nature of what they tried to verbalize. For Marie, it was when she tried to verbalize her response to vivid hallucinations by her client; while she accepted and worked with these hallucinations, it felt perhaps ephemeral, difficult to put into words: *"Well it's a bit, it's a bit … it's kind of er … it's strange"* (Marie). When analysing Stephen's interview I felt an emergent theme for him was the requirement of making his narrative 'fit', essentially looking at things in such a way that they became do-able. I felt for him, his use of words such as 'just' or 'little' seek to minimize the weight of what he is facing, thus enabling him to continue on his path without buckling at the pressure: *"After a while it's just holding a heck of a lot … So* [the potential alcohol abuse] *one little thing"* (Stephen). Dawn's narrative style was distinctive and sometimes very fluid. A fascinating extract appears to blend the client, and Dawn, in the past and present, as she endeavours to express the essence of how *she* experienced her client's powerful experience: *"And he said um 'I just put my arm out and I could feel her thigh', I can't tell you I, you know, and it lasted and did he kiss her?"* (Dawn). Similarly to Marie, Dawn also reflects verbally the struggle to place less tangible experiences within a concrete narrative structure: *"The fact there was an essence of her that he'd had yeah, and that was um yeah, well for me you know ... It was like* [laughs] *oh my God!"* (Dawn). Dawn also uses her narrative style to reflect the blunt bruising way she experienced a former supervisor: *"What the hell are you going to do? Phone the doctor? And? So what?"* (Dawn). A striking example of Lisa's use of narrative to reflect process came more from the delivery than the words. When working with clients focused on busily 'doing' after bereavement: *"*[I] *become quite calm myself and try to slow things down and calm things down with my own way of being with them really"* (Lisa). While calm and soft-toned to begin with, when delivering these words Lisa slowed down and stilled further; in that moment she *was* the process. Similarly: *"I'm quite aware of how I feel and how they feel and what's between us really"* (Lisa). This felt it succinctly contained the three element required for counselling; Counsellor, client and therapeutic relationship. Finally, Lisa is asked about the benefits of working with bereaved clients: (Whispered) *"Benefits. Mmmm"* (Lisa). An interesting feature of the subsequent answer was that, while it covers thirteen lines of transcript, a tangible expression of a benefit is only offered in the final line: *"It sort of reinforces* [that we'll sort it out together]". (Lisa). What comes before is a rundown of challenges and personal process leading to the benefit; it feels the benefit, while forming the base of the work, is not always immediately visible, hence the whisper and subsequent searching.

Master theme 3: Role of and within the Therapeutic Relationship:
The final master theme groups themes around the therapeutic relationship. I included the theme of experience in here, rather than master theme 2, because I felt that while the self of the Counsellor is affected by their experience, it is the therapeutic relationship into which the results of experience are most closely entwined.

Sub-theme 3.1: Counsellor as witness: All participants felt that they, at some point, were witness to more hidden aspects of the client, aware of what the client perhaps was not. My feeling in analysing transcripts was of their being set apart, which sits in line with the idea of Counsellors joining their clients in their journey yet remaining somehow separate. The idea of witnessing seems, at times, to aid participants in their work, such as when Stephen's feeling of being somewhat separate to his client enables him to work with their darker material without being impacted too greatly himself: *"The fact that we're holding them in that reflection … means that anything can be there. That doesn't particularly worry me … I don't find* [unconditional positive regard] *needs bounding as much, because for me it's about people's reflection of themselves"* (Stephen). Witnessing can also be a personally rewarding experience: "[His embracing of life again was] *lovely to witness, absolutely lovely"* (Dawn).

Sub-theme 3.2: The experience of experience: All participants were experienced Bereavement Counsellors. This solid grounding of experience seemed both an anchor

219

and a springboard for their work, reassuring them and allowing them more freedom to go where the client needs, as illustrated in these statements. For Lisa, it is the idea that her client's volcanic bubbling emotions: *"felt OK cos I've seen it before"* (Lisa). When Dawn considers her client's suicidal ideation she responds: *"That's quite common ... I think you get to trust yourself and the clients, so you know when you need to take action"* (Dawn). In both cases, experience seems to allow participants to hold firm for their clients. For Marie, her experience allows her to both know, and not-know, when it comes to what clients might present, illustrative of the therapist's often-paradoxical process: *"I always know that you never know what's going to happen but I know I've done it so often I've heard so many variations of the grieving process"* (Marie). Like with Dawn and Lisa, this knowledge for Marie allows her to not flinch from what clients present; her base of knowledge supporting her in her work with individual or unexpected aspects of client presentation. Lisa also found an element of professional comfort from her experience: *"So that knowledge I suppose reassured me and held me, contained me"* (Lisa). And it seems for Lisa, the client benefited from his experience of her experience too: *"I think he had a sort of respect for my knowledge and I think that held the sometimes troubled bits"* (Lisa).

Sub-theme 3.3: Relationship as 'our' tool: It felt the relationship between client and Counsellor was at times a spiralling entity; the relationship deepened because of the work undertaken, but the work was possible because of the relationship shared. These relationships are facilitative and unique, with some even creating their own language or shorthand: *"That kind of language was OK ... that's how we talked"* (Dawn). *"Sort of you know 'headless chicken' kind of thing"* (Lisa). Speaking of challenging her client, Lisa illustrates how the relationship led the work: *"Because we had the relationship then that was OK"* (Lisa). Similarly, Marie speaks of her client and how it was their relationship, and the subsequent work she did which led to her resisting labelling the client, rather than the pre-existing label dictating the style of work to begin with: *"I said she doesn't present with mental health problems ... because I found myself working from a very Person-Centred Approach"* (Marie). For Marie, the origins of the relationship are almost impossible to define: *"Somehow with her there has been a strong connection, regardless of anything, right from the very first"* (Marie). Touchingly, Dawn offers up her client to me as a gift as she closes her re-telling of their story: *"There you go, that was him. Bless him"* (Dawn).

Sub-theme 3.4: Views on the role: The final sub-theme offers participants' views on their role. This is grouped into three topics which I feel are impacted by the idea of a CG diagnosis, and a fourth general topic giving a final snapshot on what it is like to be a Bereavement Counsellor.

Sub-sub-theme 3.4.1: Suicide: Suicidal thoughts in clients are viewed by Marie as *"part I would say of every bereavement"*. Stephen also appears calm in the face of such thoughts: *"I'm not particularly concerned that a client expressing a lot of suicidal feeling is going to go out and commit suicide"* (Stephen). Both Marie and Dawn are clear on the autonomy of clients in the face of suicidal ideation: *"I deeply believe you cannot really force anybody to live, who am I to think that somebody should live, given what their life is about, yeah?"* (Marie). *"It would be his right to [commit suicide]"* (Dawn).

Sub-sub-theme 3.4.2: Nature of bereavement: The lengthy process and up-and-down nature of bereavement is illustrated by Marie and Lisa: *"But in terms of bereavement counselling* [eighteen months working together] *that's not*

221

unusual" (Marie). *"I just think that's the way grief is, comes and bites you on the bum every now and again"* (Lisa). Stephen refers to bereavement as a state – *"people in bereavement"* – while Dawn is clear on the limits of recovery in bereavement counselling: *"You can't make it better anyway can you in bereavement?"* (Dawn).

Sub-sub-theme 3.4.3: Labels: With a diagnosis of CG jarring perhaps with Person-Centred ideas, I found participants shied away from labelling: *"I was in that moment aware that as I'm working with her, I would not particularly have made that difference between 'this is complicated' or less complicated or more complicated than another … I don't like to use the word 'symptoms' but er I used to use the 'experiences' by which she expressed her present grief … Person-Centred Counselling and Complicated Grief, it is kind of, by being Person-Centred I think you open yourself up for an endless amount of complications"* (Marie). *"I get fearful of grieving being DSM defined and things like that, and being medicalised, and so even the concept of Complicated Grief, cos for me they're all unique situations"* (Stephen). *"As you can tell I'm so resistant to using that* [CG] *diagnosis"* (Dawn).

Sub-sub-theme 3.4.4: 'It's what I'm there for': The final topic seems to represent the way participants work to accept and normalize client presentations: *"For me it's um work with whatever they present … Very natural, very normal, let's normalise it"* (Dawn). *'I think it's just important um to just be where the person is … It's that sort of belief that it's OK and kind of normalising"* (Lisa). Dawn and Lisa also see their role as offering clients an ear not always accessible outside the counselling room. The final comments wrap up the overarching feelings of the second and third master themes; that the work is challenging and impactful but ultimately, this challenge links to an experiencing of purpose: *"That's a real challenge for me. But, it's what I'm there for as well … The ability to hold, to empathise with very, very powerful feelings, erm, is there as part of the job"* (Stephen).

Discussion

The findings indicated that participants sometimes underwent a duality of experience, intangible moments gained substance, images of movement offered striking insight into the experience of being in that moment, while the idea of time as linear, and thus dependable, seemed elusive. Worsley (2008) suggests that humans are complex and function psychologically at a number of levels. Participants reported examples of Worsley's 'many-layered' listening, where participants held both their concern for the client as worthy of safeguarding, and the client's phenomenological reality in equal and simultaneous regard, what Casemore (2006) refers to as attending to the whole person, and Mearns and Cooper (2005) call 'multidirectional partiality'. Duality was also found in the idea that the Counsellor may attend to a client's feeling, in line with the PCA's phenomenological underpinning (McLeod 2009), but in staying with, and using, that feeling, the Counsellor also facilitates the client through empathic process, where simply the experience of being deeply understood can be transformative (Wilkins 1999). Findings surrounding tangible and intangible ideas within the counselling process were, perhaps unsurprisingly, hard to define. For Marie there was intangibility in how she ex- perienced her client, where her language shared something of her private world (Merry 2002) as she wrestled to grasp an understanding of their process. Stephen expresses awareness that an aspect of his process works a certain way while accepting he does not clearly know the parameters of that mechanism. This ability to embrace his own positive con- victions that his awareness can be trusted, is championed by

Mearns and Thorne (2013) as central to Person-Centred Counsellors' discipline. Other examples of tangible experiencing proved impossible to reference, despite many attempts. Movement is a common image in counselling. The work is often described as a journey (Merry 2002; Mearns and Thorne 2013), and according to McLeod (2009), one aim of the PCA is to enable clients to move in the direction of their self-defined ideals. The flow of experiencing is also described (Merry 2002; McLeod 2009). However, the presumption that movement should be steady contradicts human experience (Mearns 2003). This was reflected in some images that participants used to describe their experiences of working with clients. *"Spilling"* (Stephen) and *"flooding"* (Lisa) give a flavour of the uncontainable nature of emotion and counselling work, while the *"edge"* and *"waters"* described by Marie seemed to have an air of danger about them. Lisa's *"swinging"* emotions were reminiscent of a pendulum while her reference to *"launch*[ing]*"* felt exhilarating and hopeful.

Referred to by Getsinger (1978) as the fourth dimension, the notion of time as linear development (Yariv 1999) subscribes to cultural norms of the social context in which psychotherapy takes place (Getsinger 1978). However, in keeping with the findings of this study, the complexity of psychological time renders it impossible to view as a uniform concept (Shmotkin and Eyal 2003). Stephen and Marie recalled instances where clients appeared to be experiencing the past, as if it were present, when recalling childhood abuse. Dawn's client too felt a *"current"* connection to the deceased; the immediacy of their reaction concurs with Yariv's (1999) assertion that once the consciousness of measured time is released, we are in touch with different temporal experiences. According to one study (Philippe et al. 2011), recall of autobiographical memories can influence current emotional experience. This seems supported by Dawn and Stephen when they refer to incidences which still elicit emotion in the present. Certainly, the fluid time perceptions, presented by the study, seem to confirm the supposition that perceived temporal distance is of pivotal importance (Gebauer et al. 2013) – in order to stay with the moment for clients, and ourselves, we must acknowledge internal dialogues and personal feelings (Gaudio 1998), including accepting the present impact of past events.

The findings support existing literature which indicates that the role of Bereavement Counsellor may impact on those undertaking it, bringing 'challenges and rewards on a daily basis' (Beder 2004). Positive and negative impacts were reported, along with ideas on self-care and use of narrative style to reflect process. Little is written about the benefits of being a Bereavement Counsellor (Puterbaugh 2008). Indeed, this study saw more references to negative impact on participants, than positive. However, the nature of positive gains seemed perhaps deeper and richer than their negative counterparts. The literature describes the work as a privilege (Becvar 2003), enriching (McLaren 1998), satisfying and meaningful (McLeod 2009). This level of reward is reflected in participant responses such as *"inspiring"*, *"beautiful"* and *"privilege"* (Dawn), or *"rewarding"* (Marie and Lisa). McLeod warns there is 'always more to learn' (2009, p. 653), while Merry (2002) suggests it is unhelpful for any Counsellor to consider themselves fully trained. This cycle of experience and learning seems to result in intellectual stimulation as a positive impact. Marie asks of the interaction between theory and practice, *"is there a better job?"*, and describes the work as *"intriguing"*, while Stephen calls it *"fascinating"*, and Lisa speaks of her personal learning from her client. Puterbaugh's

(2008) study suggested that Bereavement Counsellors be insightful about personal losses and attitudes to death, which Lisa's talk of *"preparing for ... sadnesses in my own life"* supports. Puterbaugh's study posits spiritual development as a feature of the work, and Dawn's *"affirming"* experiences support this. The work of counselling can also be 'highly stressful and even traumatising' (McLeod 2009, p. 653). While the essence of Person-Centred Counselling is being, not doing (Mearns 2003), it seems most Bereavement Counsellors experience feelings of helplessness (Worden 2010), inadequacy or powerlessness (Puterbaugh 2008). Dawn, Lisa and Stephen all expressed feelings of incompetence or self-questioning. This is supported by the feelings of incompetence suggested by Theriault and Gazzola (2008), described as an ongoing struggle, regardless of experience. The experience of bereavement counselling, says Puterbaugh (2008), will also touch Counsellors physically, as experienced by Marie and Lisa. Becvar (2003) suggests repeated similar experiences are cumulative in their impact, reflected by Stephen's decision to take on less complex cases. Dawn's revelation that she was *"completely oblivious to the cost"* of the work she was doing, supports Barlow and Phelan's (2007) suggestion that self-care activity is not a guaranteed outcome of knowing the importance of self-care. The centrality of self-care is widely reported in the literature, with Puterbaugh's (2008) study strongly emphasizing the need for appropriate self-care. The regular monitoring of professional practice, and physical and mental health (McLaren 1998), tending to the Counsellor's inner-self (Miller and Baldwin Jr 2013), and self-care as an ongoing process (Brady et al. 1995; Larcombe 2008; McLeod 2009; Satir 2013), seem reflected by my findings. Participants describe self-care as *"a way of living"* (Marie), *"balance"* (Dawn) or achievable through ensuring a *"good fun time outside of work"* (Lisa), the holistic self-care approach referenced by Becvar (2003). One task of supervision is the Counsellor's personal and professional development (Carroll 1996; Mearns and Thorne 2013; King 2008; McLeod 2009), and this meeting of co-professionals (Bryant-Jefferies 2006) is described by participants as *"critical"* (Stephen) and as *"reassurance"* (Dawn). However, for some participants, the support associated with self-care came from their team as much as supervision. This *"gift"* (Marie) is suggested by Barlow and Phelan (2007) as being a compelling continuous collaborative partnership, while reference is also made to the importance of groups of like-minded others (Becvar 2003; Puterbaugh 2008) for conference and support. Rennie (1998) suggests we can only understand our clients by 'living within our own experience of them' (p. 44). This was reflected by Marie and Dawn when their narrative style mirrored response; both had trouble verbally pinning down their reaction to what the client brought. This, in turn, mirrored the ephemeral nature of the clients' experiences, which in both cases could be described as hallucinatory. Narrative not only expresses but enacts (Rose and Worsley 2012), and Dawn's blunt expression of a former supervisor's attitude brings something of its bruising nature to the fore. Similarly, a striking moment has Lisa almost imperceptibly altering delivery and tone to reflect, and become the calming process she is describing. It has been suggested that our inherent capacity for language enables us to share something of our inner world with others (Merry 2002). Lisa's struggle to pinpoint tangible benefits to being a Bereavement Counsellor shows something of her inner process in balancing the weight and reward, while Stephen's use of minimizing phrases could reflect part of his process of keeping more daunting aspects of

the work at manageable levels in his narrative in order to continue.

The quality of the therapeutic relationship is often considered a core feature for counselling success (Agnew-Davies 1999; Mearns 2003; McLeod 2009; Green 2010). When the 'self' of the Counsellor, and 'self' of the client, come together to create the relationship and its outcomes (Rose 2012), it becomes a new and actively evolving entity (Aponte and Winter 2013). Participants offered insights into the unique ways in which the relationship worked for them, the impact of experience on their work within the relationship, their views on the wider sphere of bereavement counselling, and their experiences of being witness to their clients. McLeod (2009, p. 1) refers to the 'great privilege' of being witness to someone facing challenging times, a term echoed by Becvar (2003) and seemingly supported by Dawn's exclamation that seeing her client embrace life again was *"lovely to witness"*. Participants appear to be true to Rogers' (1980) definition of 'hearing' clients, in witnessing feelings and thoughts 'below the conscious intent of the speaker' (p. 8), such as the *"almost blasphemy"* heard by Marie, or *"replaying patterns"* Dawn saw. It is interesting to note for Stephen, one outcome of witnessing was increased ability to work in an *"intense and feelingful way"* (Mearns and Thorne 2013, p. 69) yet not get swamped; his witnessing takes the form of *"reflection"*, keeping focus on the client and allowing the participant to connect and join in their meaning, yet remain separate (Gaudio 1998).

All participants had worked with grief and loss for at least five years, and this base of experience appears to impact their work. It is suggested that these themes are the hardest to deal with at both professional and personal levels (Becvar 2003), and a further claim is made that aversion and discomfort associated with such work is most prevalent amongst Counsellors with little relevant training background or client contact (Kirchberg et al. 1998). It is therefore unsurprising to find these experienced Bereavement Counsellors indicating they felt *"held ... contained"* (Lisa) by their professional knowledge, or able to tolerate volatile emotion because they had *"seen it before"* (Lisa). The posture of not-knowing described by Puterbaugh (2008) and Browning (2003), is reflected by Marie's statement that *"you never know what's going to happen"*, yet she also feels comfort that she has seen *"so many variations of the grieving process"*; Marie is using her knowledge of bereaved clients to steer away from predicting behaviour, but instead to understand that behaviour once it is presented (Mearns 2003). Furthermore, Worden (2010) makes the point that novices tend to apply stage theories too literally, with Servaty-Seib (2004) concluding this may ultimately result in more complications for the client. For participants working as Person-Centred Counsellors, the primary focus could be supposed to be on the therapeutic relationship (Wilkins 1999). As a relationship between two real people, it evolves (Natiello 2001), becoming something new (Agnew-Davies 1999), as exemplified by Dawn and Lisa when they discuss the *"kind of language"* used within these unique relationships. The relationship must be solid enough to withstand challenge (Dryden 2008), and Lisa shows evidence of this in her practice when she says of challenging her client *"because we had the relationship then that was OK"*. Freedom is an important condition of the therapeutic relationship, including from diagnostic evaluation (Rogers 1961). This supports the way Marie *"found"* herself working; rather than a pre-existing label ascribed to her client dictating her style of working, she responded to what the client presented, accepting their phenomenological experiencing (Haugh 2012) and adhering to the non-directive nature of the PCA (Merry 2002). As experienced Bereavement Counsellors, participants developed their own set of philosophies around their work. Suicidal inclination is a feature of Complicated Grief (Gort 1984; Neimeyer et al. 2002; Shear 2012). A defining feature of participants' response to suicidal clients is the careful acceptance with which they receive such feelings. In keeping with their respect for client autonomy (BACP 2013), Marie felt *"you cannot really force anybody to live"*, while Dawn asserted suicide would be her client's *"right"*. Green (2010) posits it is vital suicidal clients be given space to talk about it, and Stephen seems to exemplify this therapeutic offering when he suggests he is *"not particularly concerned"* about the immediate suicide of a client expressing suicidal feelings; he is attending to process rather than outcome, suggested by both Merry (2002) and Rogers (cited in Baldwin 2013) as being facilitating at its most effective. This ability to sit with clients as they decide between life and death is also close to Rogers' (1951) idea that in being willing to allow the client to potentially choose death over life, only then can the therapist truly realize the vital strength of the individual's capacity for constructive action; in short, exhibiting deep trust in the client (Rogers 1961; Natiello 2001; McMillan 2004; Mearns and Thorne 2013), a central tenet of the PCA. Each grief response is unique (McLaren 1998) and this extends to the time support may be required. Marie suggests longer-term work is common, mentioning eighteen months as *"not unusual"*. When you consider that half the widows in the London study remained disbelieving of their loss a year on (Parkes and Prigerson 2010), the requirement for longer-term support would appear reasonable. Lisa's view is that grief re-appears at different times is reflected by the idea that people can move back and forth through grief states (Parkes and Prigerson 2010). Dawn is clear that *"you can't make it better"*, in keeping with the idea of keeping expectations realistic (Becvar 2003). A fundamental tension in this study was the tendency of the PCA to shy away from labels and work only with the client's phenomenological reality, and that CG, even of an extreme variety, can be defined as a diagnosable condition (Mearns and Thorne 2013). The participants expressed hesitation at using labels, with Dawn feeling *"so resistant"* to a CG diagnosis, and Stephen *"fearful"* of DSM definitions for grief. This hesitation to attach labels to bereavement processes is reflected in the wider literature, where there are fears this results in patholo-gizing or medicalizing grief (Shear et al. 2001; Love 2007; Simon 2012; Fox and Jones 2013). For Stephen, who says *"for me they're all unique situations"*, and Marie, who recalls *"I would not particularly have made that difference between ... complicated or less complicated"*, they seem to be simply accepting the client's phenomenological experiencing (Haugh 2012). In respecting the unique aspects of the client's grieving process (Gaudio 1998; Puterbaugh 2008), they perhaps exhibit that diminished rigidity between 'right and wrong' suggested by Natiello (2001) as a result of allowing ourselves to risk hearing another without prejudgement. In the closing topic, participants offer a snapshot of views on their role, from the normalizing of grief, suggested by Puterbaugh (2008) as often being part of the support experience, to the idea of *"work with whatever they present"* (Dawn) and being *"where the person is"* (Lisa). This idea of remaining immediate and empathically accepting of the client's phenomenology is in keeping with PCA (Merry 2002; Haugh 2012).

The sharing of grief experiences is not readily encouraged by society (Gort 1984). Another aspect of the role is, according to participants, to offer an extra dimension of support which contemporary *"society perhaps doesn't"* (Lisa). Dawn too suggests she asks the questions *"nobody else asks"*, supporting the assertion that not all Counsellors are comfortable offering bereavement counselling (Ober et al. 2012). Green (2010) suggests it can be daunting to sit with certain emotions in the counselling room. However, the ability to stay alongside clients is suggested by Stephen as *"part of the job"*. Being open to his own flow of experiencing (Merry 2002), learning from challenges (Aponte and Winter 2013) and trusting in himself as a practitioner (Natiello 2001; Mearns and Thorne 2013; Puterbaugh 2008) while retaining that solid commitment (Mearns and Thorne 2013) to clients is, simply *"what I'm there for"* (Stephen).

Conclusion

Undertaking phenomenologically based qualitative, rather than quantitative, research means I am not seeking to predict, nor to offer, generalizations in my findings (Maykut and Morehouse 1994; Willig 2008; Sanders and Wilkins 2010). Instead, the research is limited to its context, focusing on the detail of participants' process, working to a small scale, with just four participants. These participants were all from similar cultural backgrounds in that they were all white Europeans in a similar age bracket, who worked or had worked long term in a hospice environment. While generalization is not the aim of the study, more variety in the samples may have produced a different slant to the results. The specific nature of my recruitment criteria, and a tendency in Person-Centred Counsellors to shy away from labels such as CG, proved a limitation in themselves. In this vein, the lack of official definition of CG has proved a limitation to this research – even amongst the participants who replied, some clients discussed perhaps presented in ways not necessarily matching proposed CG definitions; the grief was indeed complicated, but was not necessarily Complicated Grief.

This study aimed to explore the experiences of Person-Centred Counsellors who work with clients who present with Complicated Grief, focusing on the impact on the Counsellor, and their experiences offering a Person-Centred therapeutic relationship to people grieving in this way. The outcomes indicate bereavement counselling impacted on the Counsellor's self in negative and positive ways. Awareness of pending losses, feelings of incompetence or potential burnout are some of the necessary risks while feelings of privilege, satisfaction, intellectual fulfilment and spiritual affirmation are among reported benefits. Ongoing self-care practices were suggested as central to Counsellor well-being, including supervision, team support and undertaking life-affirming activities. The study found that experience of working with the bereaved consequently provided a solid base for future bereavement work, with prior experience of grief reactions diffusing potential anxiety, allowing Counsellors to remain centred with clients' here-and-now experiences. The unique parameters of the client, Counsellor and relationship were shown to impact the process. The Counsellors displayed philosophies in keeping with Person-Centred tenets, yet potentially at odds with diagnoses such as CG, or today's frequently time-limited sessions. Suicidal inclinations were seen as common and to be respected, albeit with all possible safeguarding efforts made. Grieving was seen as an up-and-down process which may continue for years. Labels were shied away from in favour of normalizing and working with the client's reality. Finally, the study indicated the lived-experience of being in the counselling room with such clients, presented Counsellors with situations which may feel hard to pinpoint. Extreme movement is a common metaphor, chrono-logical timeframes can appear non-existent, feelings can become tangible while other knowledge can seem elusive, and both Counsellors and clients may seem to be working with two differing realities simultaneously.

Team support is cited as being beneficial to Counsellor self-care, so for lone Bereavement Counsellors, bereavement-specific peer networks may offer added layers of support. Continued attendance to self-awareness and monitoring is vital, as is ongoing training in both exploration of own-loss issues and wider issues such as specific forms of death (i.e. suicide) or issues such as child abuse or alcoholism. The experiences of being a Person-Centred Bereavement Counsellor are shown to be wide-ranging and impactful, with the self of the Counsellor directly involved, the uniqueness of grief emphasized and more intangible experiences common-place in the counselling room.

CHAPTER SEVEN

THE ROLE AND IMPACT OF THE 'MOTHER-TONGUE' IN COUNSELLING

Vida Kennedy

Introduction

I was born in North Wales in a small village into a large family. Our language at home, in the church, in the community, with my friends and at school has been Welsh, and Welsh only until I left for university aged eighteen. I learnt English aged seven and continued to study English as a subject until I was sixteen. All other subjects, including those I studied at A level, were done through the Welsh language. After leaving the North Wales area for university, I have then spent eighteen years in an English speaking environment, both at work and socially (apart from visits home to my family and friends in North Wales). In fact I have married a first language English speaker.

Although I do not feel that I have struggled academically when I shifted to predominantly speaking English, I did notice that communication in relationship, and in emotion-related aspects, were more difficult for me. Often, I found that what I was trying to say didn't come out right, or that what I was saying wasn't fully understood. This quite often left me feeling stunted and frustrated. Although I would consider myself to be a fluent and confident English speaker, there was something missing when trying to express myself in an emotional sense. I often wondered if it was a personality aspect (that is conditions of worth that I grew up with that didn't encourage talking about feelings and emotions), or could it be a language issue? My interest in this area therefore has been further fuelled by embarking on a career in Counselling. In particular my interest in the role of language in Counselling has been further increased by my client work at the Rape and Sexual Abuse Support Centre, North Wales, and from my own experience of personal therapy. A Welsh speaking client of mine often said, 'I could never have said that in English', and 'I wouldn't have been able to describe that in English'. This rang a bell with me, and indeed, for my last ten sessions of personal therapy, I chose a Welsh speaking Counsellor. I did this because I have always felt more at ease in my mother-tongue. I found my experience of personal therapy to be overwhelmingly more beneficial with my Welsh speaking Counsellor, than my previous English speaking Counsellor, and began to wonder why? The purpose of this study therefore is to increase my (and hopefully the counselling community's) understanding of the role of language, in this case, Welsh, in counselling and the counselling relationship.

My aim in this study is to explore the importance of mother-tongue in counselling. I do this in order to increase our knowledge of the issue and how it may impact on counselling and the therapeutic relationship. This will be important for those who provide counselling for Welsh speaking individuals, but also it will contribute to the wider literature on the role of mother-tongue in counselling, and may provide insights in other bilingual settings. I aimed to do this by exploring the in-depth experiences of people who consider Welsh to be their mother-tongue, and use their experiences to help me learn more about the role of their language to them, specifically in a counselling context. Therefore, my research questions were: what is the role of mother-tongue in counselling, for Welsh speaking participants? And, in what ways might it impact the counselling relationship?

In the Gwynedd county of north-west Wales, 69% of the population speak Welsh (Gathercole and Thomas 2009). In terms of the provision of quality care services, it has been said that language choice is crucial (National Assembly for Wales 2003). This fundamental aspect of care has been further highlighted by a project providing psychological services in Wales, as key in supporting Welsh individuals (Jones 2007). In a project commissioned by the Welsh Assembly, Pattison et al. (2009) describe ten recommendations for school counselling services in Wales. The seventh recommendation includes responding 'flexibly to local needs in respect of diversity (e.g. language)', and that counselling through Welsh should be made available in Welsh when 'appropriate/required' (p. 172). Although providing services through the Welsh language has been described as important (Davies 2011; Welsh Assembly Government 2012a; 2012b), I can find little research into its importance in the counselling setting. It has been said, however, that the inability of psychotherapists to speak in a client's first language can create barriers to communication between client and therapist (Verdinelli and Biever 2013; Altarriba and Santiago-Rivera 1994; Santiago-Rivera et al. 2009). It has also been described that therapeutic interventions are twice as effective when provided in a client's native language, as opposed to their second language (Griner and Smith 2006). In the literature, a person's first language has been described as the language of emotional expressiveness, and the second language associated with emotional distance (Sutton et al. 2007). The literature also suggests that language is an important aspect of the expression and processing of emotion and meaning, and on how individuals experience the world, events, and themselves (Altarriba 2003; Costa 2010; Iannaco 2009; Tehrani and Vaughan 2009). It has been said that emotional words may not always translate to another language, and that it is impossible to translate identical meaning from one language to another (Damasio 2003). In addition to these findings, the fundamental importance of language, as a means of com-municating and relating within counselling, sometimes described as 'talking therapy', has also been emphasized (Clauss 1998; Javier 1995). Such findings highlight the relevance of language in the counselling context, and further knowledge as to its role in counselling, and on the counselling relationship, will be useful to those working with Welsh speaking clients. Furthermore, it is possible that information from this study may contribute to the wider literature on the role of mother-tongue in counselling, and may provide useful insights in other bilingual settings. Welsh is a Celtic language that, although having experienced a great historical struggle for survival, has been spoken in Wales for centuries, and the 69% of Welsh speakers in Gwynedd shows its particular importance in this county. (Gathercole and Thomas 2009). Although families in Wales vary in what language they speak at home, families in which parents grew up in only Welsh speaking homes use only (96.3%), or mostly (2.8%), Welsh with their own families (Gathercole and Thomas 2009). For the purpose of this study we will use the terms 'mother-tongue' and 'first language' interchangeably, as they have been by others (Kokaliari et al. 2013). For this study, a person's mother-tongue will be seen as the language that they acquired first, and were brought up in. It is important to note, in the phenomenological spirit of this study, that we all experience things in different ways and attribute different meanings to things (McLeod 2009). For this reason, I have been open to the possibility that different persons may attribute different meanings to the above terms.

What the literature says

Language is a critical aspect of how we communicate with others. It has been described as an important aspect of our development, even before we are born, listening to sounds around us whilst in our mother's womb (Amati-Mehler et al. 1993; Maiello 1997). Early on in life, language has been described as an important aspect of the emotional attachment and relationship between mother and child (Dubinsky and Bazhenova 1997). As well as participating in our sense of belonging, language is thought to be fundamental in our separation and individualization (Bowker and Richards 2004; Hoffman 1991; Stern 1998). There are many theories on the importance of language in development (Bowker and Richards 2004; Shanahan 2008), many of which arise from a psychodynamic perspective (Bowker and Richards 2004). It is important to note, however, that from whatever perspective one considers language, its influence on development cannot be ignored. For example this study comes from a phenomenological perspective and a Person-Centred approach to counselling. Within the Person-Centred framework, the influence of the environment in which we grow has been recognized, for example, by conditions of worth (Merry 2002). Language is part of that environment, and therefore will have an influence on our development.

> Just as any unique aspect of ourselves formed during our upbringing will impact the way we relate to ourselves and the world that surrounds us, so too a bilingual's languages will differentially impact his or her interactions with the social and emotional world (Guttfreund 1990, p. 606).

Although Welsh may be a person's mother-tongue, it is crucial to point out that it exists within a bilingual setting. By the age of four and a half, most children will be speaking both Welsh and English, as both languages are taught in schools (Gathercole and Thomas 2009; Lewis 2003). The Welsh context has been described by Gathercole and Thomas (2009) as a 'stable bilingual community' (p. 216). Including Welsh within a bilingual context is important, as much of the current research with regards to the role of language in counselling comes from work with bilingual clients (e.g. Bowker and Richards 2004; Kokaliari et al. 2013; Guttfreund 1990; Javier 2007; Marcos 1976; Marcos and Urcuyo 1979; Ramos-Sanchez 2009; Santiago-Rivera et al. 2009). Bilingualism is recognized as being an important aspect in the lives of the majority of individuals around the world (Bowker and Richards 2004), and therefore it is crucial to gain further information with regards to its role in Counselling, not only for Welsh speakers, but also in other countries where bilingualism exists, especially in the current climate of increased immigration, where Counsellors might be faced with greater opportunity to work with clients where English may not be their first language.

Goncalves and Machado (2000) see emotion as crucial in understanding human change, human functioning and psychological disturbance, and therefore important within psychotherapy. Language is considered key in both accessing, and creating, emotions (in historical, social and cultural context), and therefore, if emotion is important within psychotherapy, then so is language (Lupton 1998). As discussed earlier, a person's first language has been described as the language of 'emotional expressiveness', and the second language associated with 'emotional distance' which could have implications in certain settings (Dewaele 2004; Dewaele and Pavlenko 2002; Sutton et al. 2007). Marcos (1976) and Rozensky and Gomez (1983), in particular, describe patients as more 'emotionally withdrawn' when speaking their second language. Kokaliari et al. (2013) describe it to be 'typical' for bilingual clients to switch from one language to another, returning to their mother-tongue when 'expressing strong affects, in their dreams, or when dealing with death and trauma' (p. 97). Javier (1989) also says that the more difficult an experience was, the more likely it is to be accessed using the language in which it occurred. Bilinguals are thought to switch to their first language to remember or describe emotion, and experience, in greater detail (Ramos-Sanchez 2007; Santiago-Rivera and Altarriba 2002). It has been suggested (although sometimes conflicting) that emotional words are processed differently in first and second languages of bilingual individuals (Altarriba et al. 1999; Anooshian and Hertel 1994; Sutton et al. 2007). Anooshian and Hertel (1994) conducted a recall test with Spanish-English bilingual speakers, and found that there was a higher rate of recall of emotional words in Spanish (first language) than English (second language). A different study by Altarriba et al. (1999) found that Spanish emotional words were more connected to context than their English counterparts. Emotional concepts have been seen to vary across languages, and that different languages, and word types, have different emotionality (Pavlenko 2008). Some have suggested that aspects such as the age each language was learnt; emotional context in which the language was learnt, proficiency, and nature of words (i.e. positive or negative), for example, can impact on the processing of emotional words (Harris et al. 2006; Sutton et al. 2007).

Iannaco (2009) is a psychoanalytic therapist who looked at the importance of mother-tongue where individuals have learnt a second language later on in life. He describes an extra process of 'inner translation' for bilinguals when speaking in their second language. This extra process of translation has been described to take extra effort in the process of communicating (Iannaco 2009; Imberti 2007; Marcos 1976). Furthermore, emotional words may not always translate to another language (Dewaele 2004; Dewaele 2008; Heredia and Altarriba 2001; LeDoux 1998; Sutton et al. 2007), and in fact it has been said that it is impossible to translate identical meaning from one language to another (Dewaele 2004; Damasio 2003; Iannaco 2009). The meaning of words has been said to go deeper than direct word translations (LeDoux 1998; Tehrani and Vaughan 2009), and that words are linked neurologically to memories, in which they were heard and associated with different senses and experiences, all of which are a part of creating the meanings associated to that word (Kosslyn et al. 1993). For this reason, clients have been described as switching to different languages in order to communicate what they want to say in therapy (Kokaliari et al. 2013; Santiago-Rivera et al. 2009). In fact, it has also been noted that the increased effort needed to find the right word, and/or meaning, interfered with clients' emotional expression (Marcos and Urcuyo 1979; Ramos-Sanchez 2007).

The Whorfian theory (Whorf 1950) is one of the earliest influential theories of language. This theory suggests that language impacts both thought and perception. Based on this theory others have suggested that people of different cultures and languages think and perceive things in different ways (Klineberg 1980), and that language can be a symbol of group identity (Haugen 1956). In fact, reality itself has been attached to language (de Zulueta 1990, 1995). This phenomenon has been described by Ervin (1964) as a shift from one way of being to another, when changing from one language to another. This shift has also been described by others, whereby language is linked to the context in which it was learnt, and that this context is attached to a particular set of attitudes, values, and associations.

> Mother-tongue, as it is called, will be the one in which a child's early years will be enveloped. This mother-tongue will most likely be associated with a particular set of thoughts and feelings. The child's associations will depend on the experiences per se (Guttfreund 1990, p. 604).

Burck (1997) says that 'different languages encompass different world views, which makes it understandable that bilingual persons report that they have very different experiences in different languages' (p. 71). It has also been suggested that a person may experience different aspects of the self in different languages, and therefore the existence of dual self or dual identity (Altarriba 2003; Amati-Mehler et al. 1993; Burck 2004; Marcos and Urcuyo 1979; Perez-Foster 1996; Tehrani and Vaughan 2009; Tummala-Narra 2001). Perez-Foster (1996) describes bilinguals as living in a 'dual-reality' (p. 99). Greenson (1950) was one of the first to describe the existence of different identities in different languages. He described a bilingual patient who when speaking German, felt like a 'scared, dirty, child', and whilst speaking English, felt like a 'nervous, refined woman' (Bowker and Richards 2004, p. 464). This idea of dual identity may be supported by other descriptions of how different languages come with different emotional and cultural dimensions (Altarriba and Santiago-Rivera 1994; Altarriba and Soltano 1996; de Zulueta

1995). Drawing on Hoffmann's (1991) work, Bowker and Richards (2004) say: 'National identity as well as self-identity can be very strongly rooted in the maintenance of a particular language' (p. 463). Tehrani and Vaughan (2009) describe how each language allows a person to show and experience different aspects of the self. This importance of language in identity, may be particularly relevant to Welsh clients. Giles et al. (1974) describe language as the most important dimension of ethnic identity for Welsh individuals. Although their sample was small for a quantitative study, it remains one of the few studies into the role of the Welsh language in Welsh identity. More recently, a study by Livingstone et al. (2009) has supported their findings.

Bilingual clients are said to switch from one language to the other during therapy (Kokaliari et al. 2013). Psychoanalytical work with bilingual clients has dominated the platform from which we learn about language in therapy. Early psychoanalysts, such as Buxbaum (1949) and Greenson (1950), describe how bilingual clients used their second language within therapy as a means of defence (although unconsciously) against the emergence of repressed fantasies or difficult feelings. Therefore, using a second language was used to create emotional distance in therapy (Bowker and Richards 2004). The work of Buxbaum (1949) suggested that effective therapy is not possible when a therapist does not speak the clients' language, that if experiences are encoded within a certain language, they cannot be accessed in the same way by another. Others such as Marcos and Alpert (1976), however, say that there is no evidence to support this. The role of language in creating closeness, and/or distance, remains of great importance within Counselling. Whether seen as a negative or positive aspect of therapy, the idea that language can influence access to emotional reactions, and act as a defence against painful material, has been supported by many (e.g. Burck 2004; Costa 2010; Damasio 2003; Kokaliari et al. 2013; Kosslyn et al. 1993; LeDoux 1998; Marian and Neisser 2000). This aspect of language (creating distance) in therapy relates to safety. Safety is often described as an important aspect of creating an effective environment for therapy (Merry 2002). There are those who describe the use of mother-tongue in therapy as an aspect of creating a safe and trusting environment (e.g. Damasio 2003; LeDoux 1998; Marian and Neisser 2000; Tehrani and Vaughan 2009; Sprowls 2002). Gilbert (2005) suggests that a child who is exposed to physical and verbal soothing, develops an enhanced self-soothing neuro-pathway. This suggests that the language you were soothed in as a child will act as a soother later on in life. There is, however, more to this than meets the eye. Tehrani and Vaughan (2009) describe a case study of a therapeutic process of a bilingual lady who had experienced bullying. The study supports the idea that language is crucial in accessing the emotions related to an event. It describes that 'the full intensity of the traumatic experience had been lost in the translation' (p. 13). Although it suggests that this acts as a barrier to accessing the felt emotions, the therapist here saw it as beneficial, because 'on this occasion it appeared that the dilution of the emotional response to translation of the trauma story was helpful, as it assisted in the narrative re-trieval without triggering the emotional response held in the preconscious trauma memory' (p. 13). Caution in using mother-tongue to access traumatic experiences has also been highlighted by others (e.g. Paradis 2008). Sprowls (2002) described that therapists switch to the clients' first language, to create a safe environment and access deeper emotions, but then switch to the clients' second language to help them distance themselves when emotions become too powerful.

Language has also been described as something that can create closeness or distance within the therapeutic relationship. Bowker and Richards (2004), for example, describe how, in their qualitative study of therapists working in English with bilingual clients, they found that participants felt varying degrees of distance and separation from their clients. They described needing to pay extra attention to communication aspects to make a good connection with their clients. Santiago-Rivera et al. (2009) found that switching to their clients' first language was used to increase communication, connection, trust and bonding in the re-lationship. Kokaliari et al. (2013) also described language as an important factor for creating a therapeutic alliance. The participants in their study described issues of trust, idealization and hostility towards the psychotherapist. Transference and countertransference within psychotherapy has been discussed in the literature with relation to language. The language of clients and therapists has been linked to associations of historical and cultural perceptions, awareness and prejudices, and that this may impact the therapeutic relationship via transference and countertransference (Comas-Diaz and Jacobsen 1991). Possible results have been described to include mistrust, hostility, lying, idealization, and power issues (Comas-Diaz and Jacobsen 1991; Kokaliari et al. 2013). Further information can be found elsewhere (e.g. Clauss 1998; Comas-Diaz and Jacobsen 1991; Kokaliari et al. 2013; Perez-Foster 1998). This issue may be worth considering in this study due to the historical struggle for power and language that exists between the Welsh and English (Livingstone et al. 2009). Findings, with regards to impact of therapist ethnicity on therapy effectiveness, are mixed (Ramos-Sanchez 2009; Verdinelli and Biever 2013). Clients whose therapist language and ethnicity match, however, have been found to be more satisfied and less likely to drop out (Campell and Alexander 2002; Griner and Smith 2006). More importantly, interventions done in a person's native language, have been found to be twice as effective as those in their non-native language (Griner and Smith 2006). What has been made clear so far, is that when it comes to working with bilingual clients, it is considered beneficial for the therapist to be aware of aspects related to bilingualism that can impact therapy (Clauss 1998; Kokaliari et al. 2013). For example, that clients can use language as a defence against painful material (Buxbaum 1949; Bowker and Richards 2004; Kokaliari et al. 2013). Costa (2010) learns from bilingual therapists, and suggests being aware of clients' linguistic history, expression of emotions differently in different languages, impact of language on identity and culture, how meaning is conveyed, and how it relates to people's experiences of learning, and how speaking in a second language can be helpful for therapists working with bilingual clients. Language is how clients and therapists connect (Kokaliari et al. 2013), and therefore, it will be crucial in the therapeutic relationship. It should be noted that much of the above research is based upon psychodynamic approaches, *none* of which focus specifically on the case of Welsh speakers or on the Person-Centred approach to Counselling. This highlights a large gap in knowledge with regards to the role of Welsh (as a mother-tongue) in Person-Centred Counselling and the counselling relationship.

Participants

For this study, purposive (non-probability) sampling was adopted where participants are selected in accordance with the needs of the study (Denscombe 2014; Strang 2000). This allowed for accessing individuals with particular relevance to the research topic. Criteria for inclusion included: being over the age of eighteen; speaking Welsh as their first language/ mother-tongue; having experienced counselling; being Counsellors or trainee Counsellors who have access to supervision to ensure that they have the necessary support; being individuals who are not Counsellors and have been out of therapy for two years. The goal of these criteria was to ensure that my participants had experience in the area of interest, and to ensure minimal risk for distress through participation. Placement of posters was used to gain maximum access to the target population, including local universities with access to Welsh speaking students; and also organizations offering counselling services in Welsh speaking areas. All documents were available in Welsh. Four participants volunteered for the study. All four participants were female, and were either trained, or in-training, Counsellors. All currently lived in the North Wales area. All four participants have been given pseudonyms for confidentiality reasons.

The first participant, Gwenno, aged thirty-one, was a qualified Person-Centred Counsellor working within North Wales. She described her background, current work, social, and family settings, as being predominantly Welsh. She described Welsh as both her mother-tongue and first language from the outset, and described throughout her interview difficulties in expressing herself (even in the interview) in English. She had experienced Person-Centred

Counselling through the medium of English, although she described the majority of her current work as a therapist to be through the medium of Welsh.

The second participant, Sian, aged thirty-two, was a trainee Person-Centred Counsellor, currently in her second year at a university in England. She described her background, current working, social and family settings, as being predominantly Welsh speaking. She is currently living in North Wales. She described Welsh as both her mother-tongue and first language from the outset. She had and is experiencing Person-Centred Counselling through the medium of Welsh. She has also, however, experienced some English counselling settings at university, e.g. triad work.

The third participant, Ffion, aged thirty-three, was a trainee Person-Centred Counsellor, currently in her third year at a university in England. She described having a predominantly Welsh upbringing until the age of sixteen, but then described living and working in an English environment, and becoming more confident in speaking English than Welsh, although she still describes Welsh as both her mother-tongue and her first language. She has recently moved back to North Wales and now most of her working and social contexts are Welsh. She had, and is experiencing, Person-Centred Counselling through the medium of Welsh. However, in the past she has experienced counselling through the medium of English and in some English counselling settings at university. In addition she has started a counselling placement in Wales, and has experienced being the Counsellor in both Welsh and English.

The fourth participant, Cadi, aged sixty-six, is a fully qualified Person-Centred Counsellor, who has been working as a Counsellor in both English and Welsh settings. She currently lives in North Wales. However, she has lived away from Wales for the majority of her life since leaving for university. Although initially describing Welsh as her first language and mother-tongue, during the interview she then described that actually by now her first language is probably English, although her mother-tongue is still Welsh. She currently feels most comfortable speaking English. She has always had her own counselling through the medium of English, but does offer counselling to others through the medium of Welsh.

Data collection

This study employed semi-structured interviews for data collection as this style of interviewing allows the participant to talk about what is important to them, as well as allowing the researcher to have a schedule of topics to discuss that are related to the research interests. The interview schedule consisted of the following questions:

- What would you consider to be your first language or mother-tongue, and what does that mean to you?
- Please could you tell me a little about when you learned your first and second language, and the context in which you have developed and used both.
- How comfortable would you say do you feel speaking in both your first and second language?
- What aspects did you consider important in choosing your therapist?
- How important was the language of your therapist in your decision?
- What was your reasoning behind choosing an English speaking or Welsh speaking therapist?

- Having received counselling, how important do you think language was/is in your therapy and/or relationship with your Counsellor?
- Were some things easier to talk about in Welsh than in English, or the other way around?
- Were some emotions easier or harder to express in a particular language?
- Were some words more difficult to explain/describe in one language or the other? Did you feel that what you meant was always understood? And that you could always express what you meant?
- Do you feel the same when you talk Welsh, as when you talk English?
- Do you experience things the same, or differently, depending on the language that it is experienced?
- Do you think culture and language are linked, and if so, how important is this when communicating with your therapist?
- What is your attitude towards speaking English/English speakers?
- Do you think that being Welsh influenced how your personal therapist interacted with you/perceived you?
- How important do you think language is in your relationships? In particular with your Counsellor?
- Can you describe any difficulties or benefits related to language in your therapy?
- Do you feel self-conscious, or less confident, when speaking English with a Counsellor (or with other professional people)?
- For those who have experiences of counselling in both languages, and if not described in the above questions,

how would you compare your experience of receiving counselling in Welsh and English?

- Having experienced counselling, if you were looking for a Personal Therapist in the future do you think that what language they spoke would play a role in whom you chose?

All interviews were conducted in English due to no Welsh speaking examiners being available at the University of Chester.

Findings

A breakdown of the master themes and sub-themes is shown in Table 11.

Theme number	Master theme name	Sub-ordinate themes
1	Access to Feelings, Emotions, and Experiences	1.1 Familiarity 1.2 Identity and culture 1.3 Flowing from within (natural)
2	Getting in the Way of Therapy	2.1 Thinking and finding the words 2.2 Feeling misunderstood
3	Creating a Trusting and Facilitative Relationship with the Counsellor	3.1 Pre-existing connection and bond 3.2 Acceptance 3.3 Safety 3.4 Understanding
4	Extras that Come with Having Two Languages	4.1 Choice and flexibility 4.2 Hidden issues

Table 11: Table of master and sub-ordinate themes identified.

Master theme 1: Access to Feelings, Emotions and Experiences
  Sub-theme 1.1: Familiarity: All participants described
the language they were currently most familiar with, as the
easiest language to communicate about their feelings,
emotions and experiences. For Gwenno and Sian, they both
described Welsh as the language they were most familiar
with, used in all aspects of their lives, and felt more confident
using. It allowed them more effortless access to their emotions
than when they spoke a less familiar second language: *"My
emotions would be easier in Welsh. Erm ... it's just what's in you
really, isn't it? And what you know and what you've always spoken,
I suppose. And it's just, erm ... more real isn't it, I think. Personal
things and personal emotions and feelings and thoughts are more
real and here and now and it would be better or easier to do that in
Welsh really"* (Gwenno). *"... during sort of heightened emotion
and maybe, you know, really expressing feeling and doing that
easily without having the risk of not remembering words and all that
type of things that ... I think it's very, very important that people
are able to do that in their mother-tongue"* (Sian). Cadi describes
her younger years as being Welsh speaking, but then as she
grew and moved away from Wales, English became easier for
her. *"Welsh is my first language. I was brought up in a very rural
... on a farm. I obviously learnt English in school when I was about
... when I was eight onwards. But, I must say, I do feel more
comfortable in English now ... I suddenly switch to English when I
want to say what I want to say, you know, something a bit deeper"*
(Cadi). For Ffion, it is less clear cut. Although she described
speaking Welsh as easier for her when she was younger, her
more English-based educational history and development
changed to her feeling more comfortable speaking English.
Unlike Cadi, however, since her return to Wales, not all of her
experiences continue to be easier in English. Although
personal and deeper emotions are easier in English, those

experiences that occurred within a Welsh speaking context were easier for her to talk about in Welsh. *"I think maybe sometimes things to do with my relationship, because my partner's Welsh and, you know, all our interactions, all our connections are in Welsh language. It makes sense to me, it seems easier to talk about that in Welsh. Erm ... whereas, maybe stuff that's to do with myself, the way I feel about myself and some of those other ... sort of, maybe more hidden things. That feels like it's easier in English. Like an internal/external thing almost"* (Ffion). The most currently familiar language appears to be easier for communicating emotions and deeper issues, and therefore language is important. It also, however, describes that this language may not always be what the individual considers to be their mother-tongue, and that context, as well as familiarity, may have a role to play in which language is easier for communicating.

Sub-theme 1.2: Identity and culture: Language seems to play an important role within the participants' identity and culture, and therefore in how they see and express themselves. The participants describe how what language they speak can provide an insight into who they are as a person, and where they came from. Gwenno, for example, describes how being Welsh and speaking Welsh is part of who she is, and maybe if she is not speaking Welsh, she is not being herself. *"I feel different. I feel me, I suppose, when I speak Welsh. It feels comfortable. I'm able to express myself clearly. It's, you know, natural. I feel more confident"* (Gwenno). She also describes the importance of her therapist understanding what being Welsh means, and what the culture involves, in order to feel understood as a person. Below, Sian also describes how understanding her culture gives an understanding of who she is. *"Welsh culture's a very important part of who I am, my family,* *my friends, you know, the fact that, you know, you're a minority I suppose. Erm ... and I suppose ... I suppose, with regards to the therapist, what I would want, always, is that there would always be understanding there"* (Sian). Ffion (and also Gwenno and Sian) sees the Welsh language as a part of who she is, a part that cannot be explained – only felt. And this again is linked to how unless she can explain, or feel understood, then *she,* as a person, cannot be fully understood. *"... because it is **so** integral to who I am and how I see myself in the world. It's not something that I'm always aware of myself. And so to explain that to someone else ... it's like me asking an English person 'what does it mean to you to be speaking English?' It's just ... it just is, you know"* (Ffion). In addition to being a part of who she is, it also impacts on her personality. She describes how she is more formal when speaking English, but more *"friendly and jokey"* when speaking Welsh. For Cadi, however, although being Welsh, and speaking Welsh was part of her younger identity, she doesn't see it as part of her adult identity. In fact, she feels more in tune with English culture. *"I suppose I've lived in England for so long I've become half English really. And I've lived in America as well. So I don't feel Welsh any more, and when I came back here, I had counselling because I couldn't settle because I didn't feel that I belonged"* (Cadi). For Gwenno, Sian, and Ffion, speaking Welsh is part of feeling as if they belong, and part of expressing their identity and feeling fully understood as a person. For Cadi, however, speaking Welsh does the opposite – it makes her feel as if she doesn't belong, and it doesn't give understanding of who she is now as a person.

Sub-theme 1.3: Flowing from within (natural): This theme has close links to the above two themes, but describes how communicating about emotions and feelings is impacted by where the information is coming from. Familiarity may come with practice or fluency. However, there is an element of speaking about emotions and personal issues that comes from a deeper place. Gwenno, for example, describes speaking Welsh as something that feels natural, and that happens without effort as if it flows out of her when she speaks Welsh. *"I think it just comes natural in your first language doesn't it? It's something ... erm ... it's your first language and it's just natural and it just happens and you're able to express yourself I think better, maybe ..."* (Gwenno). A similar phenomenon is described by Sian, where it feels more instinctive and natural. *"I find it easier talking in my mother-tongue compared to if I'm speaking in English, for example. And it seems to be more ... Yeah, I suppose instinctive. And, there's less effort involved too, I suppose when I speak in Welsh, compared to when I speak in English"* (Sian). Ffion seems to describe aspects of herself that cannot be accessed through English – a place that feels deep within her soul. *"But then there's that aspect of speaking Welsh where there are certain things that I just can't say in English. It sort of comes from somewhere else almost"* (Ffion). Cadi, on the other hand, although describing a part of her deep inside as being Welsh, she doesn't feel it is inaccessible through English. *"I do feel more in touch with my ground and my being, I suppose, in Welsh. But it doesn't really count for that much really, because of all my developments since I was five say. You know, there is an area, I suppose, deep inside me somewhere which is a little Welsh girl, you know, five years old who stood on the chair to speak in English, you know. But really, I don't have ... to talk in Welsh to access that little girl really, even though she's Welsh"* (Cadi).

Master theme 2: Getting in the Way of Therapy
For the participants in this study there were elements of language that got in the way of therapy, or allowed therapy to feel successful. This master theme describes areas in which

256

therapy was impeded and/or facilitated by the language used.

Sub-theme 2.1: Thinking and finding the words: In the above theme of familiarity, we have seen that how familiar or comfortable the participants feel with a language can impact upon how easy it feels to communicate within therapy; a more specific aspect of this familiarity that has been described as having an impact on therapy is that of searching for words. Gwenno describes how her difficulty in searching for the right word can act as a barrier to exploring the issues she needs to explore. *"And I suppose, I think in Welsh first as well. So I think and then I'd speak Welsh wouldn't I, really what I was thinking. So ... it would maybe stop things as well I suppose ... with ... because there's so many distractions isn't there? Thinking and translating maybe, or ... a lot of thinking before saying something really. And that maybe has affected the session in the way of what I was going to talk about maybe"* (Gwenno). Sian describes how searching for the words can impact the counselling session, because it blocks access to how she is feeling and, in fact, changes the feeling from what she was trying to explain to that of frustration. *"I'm so busy trying to find particular words, that actually how I'm feeling – the emotions and feelings actually get lost in the process of searching, I suppose, which can be quite frustrating"* (Sian). For Ffion, she describes some particular words, relevant to counselling, easier in English, therefore not being able to access these words in Welsh can be a barrier for her. *"I don't know what, you know, Person-Centred therapy even would be in Welsh particularly"* (Ffion). Cadi describes a similar problem with Welsh. This was more unexpected, as there is little written about those who have difficulty speaking what they themselves describe as their mother-tongue. She feels that searching for Welsh words can feel like a *"chore"*, and this could act as a barrier in therapy. *"I wouldn't know how to express some deep words in Welsh without having to look in the dictionary. And then it becomes a chore really"* (Cadi). Therefore, searching for words and thinking, have been described as aspects that can interfere with the process, with the flow of the counselling session. It can be distracting, frustrating, tiresome, and it can take away the immediacy of it. A strong theme described by the participants was one connected to how language can impact on the meaning of what they want to say. Gwenno describes her struggle in feeling that what she is saying is what she means. *"What I noticed with words, they're not quite the same. Erm ... so maybe translating an emotion or a word – feeling word or something – isn't quite the same to what I was trying to express, if that makes sense. Maybe they are the same words, but they don't mean the same. Erm ... that's quite hard to explain as well really. The meaning, I suppose, is different. Or, to me, it feels different. I suppose if I can't get that meaning across to what I feel or think, it's not quite the same ... it goes back to the ... me not being able to express the right feeling, maybe, or not getting that across to what it actually really does feel or mean to me"* (Gwenno). For Sian, a problem is that she doesn't feel that the gravity that comes with a particular word in Welsh gets carried with its English translation. *"... obviously, you know, you've got a range of words to describe sadness, but it's that extremity of it maybe that maybe gets lost sometimes"* (Sian). Ffion describes a similar phenomenon, where there are some words that carry so much meaning in Welsh, but not in English, and how this can have an effect on the impact a word has on you. *"She will be speaking in English and a little bit of Welsh creeps in and she'll say one word and it's like something has hit you, like a stake through your heart. It's just so ... packed with meaning"* (Ffion). Cadi, however, although she recognizes there are some words that do not have a direct translation, doesn't feel that this causes any problems for her. *"Apart from something like 'hiraeth' which is the obvious one. You know, and there might be one or two words, but they're just the same in any language. You can't quite translate them,* (and did you think that that impacted you at all?) *Not at all! Not at all"* (Cadi).

Sub-theme 2.2: Feeling misunderstood: This theme is closely linked to the above theme about loss of meaning. This theme, however, focuses more on how not being able to get across what something means to you, or how you are feeling (feeling misunderstood) can impact the counselling session. Gwenno, for example, describes it as frustrating. *"… not being able to explain myself properly maybe, or the counsellor not getting what I was trying to say or whatever. So frustrating I think more than anything"* (Gwenno). Sian describes it as confusing, where the confusion she already feels inside can be amplified by the confusion of feeling misunderstood, and not being able to get across what is going on with her: *"… because I've got it here in Welsh, but I'm trying to work out, maybe sometimes, what it is in English. And maybe the therapist will pick up on something, but that's not really what I'm saying, but there's confusion within me anyway, so it's sort of … it can be quite confusing"* (Sian). For Ffion, because the weight of what she is trying to say has not been understood, she feels dismissed, without a voice. *"… it does have a direct translation, but it meant more to me – the Welsh word. It was 'blaguro'. It's like everything was blossoming … Erm … budding, and sort of full of potential. And I remember saying it in the group [laughter] and just, you know. I knew they understood, but I did feel a little bit dismissed maybe"* (Ffion). On the other hand, Cadi has never experienced feeling misunderstood, and felt her Counsellor got exactly what it was she was trying to say, and that this felt good (tone of voice) *"… and she asked me about my childhood, which suddenly … just went straight there,*

259

and I described it to her – on a Welsh farm, you know. And she just got it, immediately" (Cadi).

Master theme 3: Creating a Trusting and Facilitative Relationship with the Counsellor

Sub-theme 3.1: Pre-existing connection and bond: This theme focuses on how having a Welsh speaking therapist can be seen as a having a head start in the relationship building aspect of counselling, because of the feeling that there is already a level of understanding from the outset; that there is something connecting the client and the Counsellor before they even begin. Gwenno describes how this understanding allows the relationship to go further. *"I think there's maybe a deeper understanding. I wouldn't say better. There's sort of a deeper understanding of each other in the relationship and in the counselling process. I think it helps or it adds to the relationship a lot, to build on the relationship and go further really"* (Gwenno). Sian and Ffion also describe the importance of feeling understood, and how it creates a bond between them and their therapist from the start. *"... it's like being in tune with someone. So, it's that sort of, really feeling, yeah, in tune and being understood from the offset, I suppose"* (Sian). *"People that maybe are from Wales or do speak Welsh, you know, there's a natural connection there anyway"* (Ffion). Ffion (as does Gwenno and Sian) also describes how it relates to culture and identity, and the importance of having shared-experiences that create a bond between client and Counsellor. *"... if I was to talk about experiences of going to Eisteddfod as a child, no one else would understand what that entailed or what it means or, you know, just certain life event sort of things, that happen. You know, I was able to share everything like that with her and all these different words and things that meant stuff to me, that I couldn't have done"* (Ffion). Although Cadi doesn't feel the need for this understanding in her own counselling, she does recognize its existence, and how important it is for other Welsh speakers. *"... when they knock on the door and they say 'Oh, you know, I'm Jane', and I say 'Dewch I mewn da chi isho panad', or something, and I can see them visibly relaxing, and I think a lot of work is done in that very moment, you know, by the fact that I'm ... and you know, I've got quite a local accent really. I can ... They can think 'Oh right, she's not one of them, you know, anonymous, Ysbyty G (local hospital) people'"* (Cadi).

Sub-theme 3.2: Acceptance: This theme relates to a strong feeling that if a person accepts the Welsh language and culture, then they feel accepted as a person. Furthermore, a sense of their struggle with language difficulties being accepted, feels important for the relationship. For Gwenno, the fact that her struggle was understood and accepted, actually helped the relationship. *"I wouldn't refuse to see somebody because they weren't Welsh speaking. It's just that understanding or knowledge and acceptance I suppose which, you know, I received which helped the process"* (Gwenno). Sian also highlights the importance of having a therapist who understands the importance of Welsh in her life, and that this contributes to feeling accepted as a person. *"Welsh culture's a very important part of who I am, my family, my friends, you know, the fact that, you know, you're a minority I suppose. With regards to the therapist, what I would want, always, is that there would always be understanding there"* (Sian). In addition, for Ffion, is the perception that people may be prejudiced to the Welsh, and therefore to her, and how this could result in her closing down. *"I do feel like sometimes I am perceived negatively because, just as, you know, people carry prejudices of different things – I know there's some people that are quite anti-Welsh ... I know that's their issue, but then that makes me feel, sort of, closed down, like I don't have a voice then"* (Ffion). For Cadi, acceptance is important, but is experienced in a different way. She describes not feeling accepted within her Welsh relationships, and therefore feels greater acceptance within an English context. *"But I can see it's a sensitive point, you know, that my children don't speak English because they were brought up in England, you know. But we get on fine, but there's that little thing there. 'Why don't your children speak English – Welsh?'"* (Cadi).

Sub-theme 3.3: Safety: This focuses on how language can be used as a message of safety and in the development of trust between client and Counsellor. For Gwenno, the feeling of safety is closely linked to familiarity and comfort. *"Erm ... feels comfortable, safer, **clearer** really. It just feels better and safe and more comfortable to, for me anyway, to speak it. Because that's the language I've been brought up with really, isn't it, and that's I think the reason, but, definitely, I feel more ... (pause) ... more me. More myself, speaking it"* (Gwenno). Sian describes how language can be used as a tool to manage how safe she feels when talking about different issues. If it becomes unsafe, she can always switch to English, which can create a distance between her and a painful issue. *"I suppose if you want a bit of distance from something, I sometimes find it easier doing that in English. So, if I'm trying to distance myself somehow, for whatever reasons, erm ... then sometimes it's easier to do that in English compared to Welsh. So really, when I'm trying to get really close to something, I find it easier doing that in Welsh"* (Sian). For Ffion, it is an important aspect of the relationship development and trust, enabling her to feel safe. For Cadi, although she doesn't describe feeling safer using Welsh herself, she does describe it as an important aspect of offering safety to her own Welsh speaking clients. *"I meet people for initial meetings or counselling if they want it in Welsh, and I can see the relief on their face when I say 'do you want a panad (cup of tea)', or something in Welsh. And I think that's a huge thing for them. I can tell! And I like giving that* *to them and I speak to them in Welsh then"* (Cadi). For Cadi, it may be that actually speaking English feels safer for her, because she does describe negative associations and past experiences within a Welsh context, suggesting that language is related to safety for Cadi too.

Sub-theme 3.4: Understanding: This theme has a strong link to the above themes of pre-existing connection and acceptance, but also to the master theme 'Getting in the way of therapy'. It focuses on how feeling understood by their therapist is crucial to the relationship, and therefore to therapy. Gwenno is left feeling frustrated and disappointed when she doesn't feel understood by her therapist. *"Disappointing, yes. That's the word, really. Erm ... trying to get something across or trying to really explain something and knowing maybe that the other person or the counsellor doesn't understand"* (Gwenno). Sian has described how being 'stunted' in searching for words can impact the relationship, but further than this, it can cause a problem in feeling that the therapist understands what it is she is trying to say *"... because I maybe don't get to that particular word, that then the therapist picks up on something which I'm not really getting at"* (Sian). It can also cause difficulties with regards to understanding from the client's side. Ffion, for example, felt she misunderstood what to expect from therapy, which impacted her experience negatively. *"But there was a language problem in that there was a miscommunication, erm ... in terms of what was provided to me and what I knew of the service and my expectation, and all that sort of thing"* (Ffion). What is important for the client, is that what they feel, that what they are trying to say, is understood. For the above three, this isn't always the case when speaking English. For Cadi, however, it is just as important that what she is trying to say is understood, but for her, language has not been a barrier to this.

Master theme 4: Extras that Come with Having Two Languages

Sub-theme: Choice and flexibility: Having a choice was an important issue described by all; the importance of having a choice themselves and/or being able to offer this choice to others. Gwenno, for example, felt disappointed by the lack of choice she had in choosing the right therapist for her. *"So, there wasn't a choice really, either. So that's ... that was a frustration before starting the process, if that makes sense?"* (Gwenno). Having a choice of languages has been described as allowing flexibility with regards to staying close to, or creating distance from issues. Sian and Ffion highlight this below: *"So, if I'm trying to distance myself somehow, for whatever reasons, erm ... then sometimes it's easier to do that in English compared to Welsh. So really, when I'm trying to get really close to something, I find it easier doing that in Welsh"* (Sian). *"And, at one point, I know the, sort of, first four sessions really, I was able to use that (using the Welsh formal 'chi' for you) as an excuse and not get close and to sort of avoid painful things"* (Ffion). Having more than one language available can be seen as a positive when it comes to therapy. For example, Ffion and Cadi suggest further options of exploration when there is more than one languages available. *"But, erm ... I would like to have a choice of, erm ... language. And I think actually, I would choose a Welsh counsellor just because then you've got more options, because I can change and throw in an English word or an English sentence if I need to, but I don't have that freedom if it's just a single language counsellor. So I think I would, yeah. It would be important"* (Ffion). *"I'm aware that people who are bilingual do have a slightly easier time of it because they've got the two ways of expressing things really. You* *know, that's ... yeah. Two different cultures to work things through in"* (Cadi).

Sub-theme 4.2: Hidden issues: For all participants, the presence of more than one language in their lives allowed for discovery, and/or exploration, of unique hidden issues. For Gwenno, a hidden issue was her lack of confidence in speaking English. She was able to identify this and explore it openly with her therapist, which she found to be a beneficial aspect of her therapy. For Sian, this hidden issue was in regards to the difficulties she experienced working in a small rural setting. *"The only disadvantage, but then again, I'm not sure if this is down to language, is the awareness that I have with my therapist that she may know the people that I work with and ... So, there's a sense of, because we're a minority language and that we live in a very small place, there's that risk of, you know, they may know who I'm talking about. And then, because there's that risk, maybe I ... Maybe I hold back a bit about what I say and how I say it in case that person knows"* (Sian). For Ffion, it seemed as if there were many hidden issues related to language. One of the most prominent issues, I felt, was the inner conflict that she had with the historical part of her, to which Welsh was so very important, and the more recent part of her that felt most comfortable in English. This seemed to bring out feelings of guilt and betrayal. Because she may not be as 'Welsh' as she would like to be, demonstrating the hold that being Welsh has on her and her identity. *"... it's strange as well because then I've got this, sort of, historical side of me that is almost sad that there's been that change as I've grown up, because it does mean so much. You know, because I've never ... I could never imagine my children for example not being able to speak Welsh or them not going to a Welsh school. And as I've grown up, (...) so there is a huge part of me that still wants to have that in my life and to, you know, really I would like to be as comfortable talking about myself in Welsh"*

(Ffion). For Cadi as well, there seems to be a hidden issue about what Welsh means to her. Often she associates Welsh with being backwards, bad experiences, having limits and being judged. English, however, is associated with freedom, culture, and acceptance. Although each participant may have discovered a different hidden issue, it appears to be that if it wasn't for the presence of two languages, that issue may never have come to light.

Discussion

This study has identified several aspects of mother-tongue that may be considered important for counselling and the counselling relationship, and that these aspects can influence how effective the counselling will be for individuals. The familiarity of the client with the language used in counselling, has been described as having a role in determining how easy it is for individuals to access, and talk about, emotions, personal issues and experiences. The more familiar a client is with a language the easier it will be to access such aspects. Furthermore, the study describes that a person's identity and culture can be linked to mother-tongue, and that this can influence how they express themselves and believe them-selves to be understood, and accepted, by others, including the therapist. Where a person feels that their therapist has knowledge of their language and culture they feel that they have a more complete knowledge of who they are as a person. The study also highlights specific areas related to language that can cause difficulties in the counselling context. Examples of these include: difficulties searching for words when the client is speaking in a language other than their mother-tongue or first language (English in this case); and difficulties in expressing the exact meaning of what they are feeling, or trying to say, due to not having direct translations available, or words having different meanings in Welsh and English. These issues can impact on the counselling process and on how an individual feels within counselling, in particular with regards to feeling understood. The study describes how language plays a role in the counselling relationship, by contributing towards trust and acceptance, as well as feeling safe within the counselling relationship. The bilingual aspect of these participants (being able to speak Welsh and English) described as creating 'extra' issues that may not be relevant for mono-lingual clients, and that these issues are important to be aware of. For example, how clients can manage how close to, or distant, from an issue they keep themselves by choosing what language to use in therapy, and how having formal and informal ways of addressing others can impact the counselling session and relationship. Finally, the study also uses the idiopathic nature of the study methodology as a way of highlighting the individual nature of the role of language for clients in therapy, and how being aware of these issues can be helpful for clients and therapists.

The findings suggest that language plays an important role in counselling and in the counselling context. This supports findings of others (e.g. Clauss 1998; Costa 2010; Iannaco 2009; Santiago-Rivera and Altarriba 2002; Tehrani and Vaughan 2009) – all of whom suggest that language is important in counselling, in particular with regards to accessing emotions and experiences that were gained within a particular language context. Firstly, the findings suggest that what language you use within counselling can impact access to emotions, and personal aspects and experiences. Dewaele (2004), Dewaele and Pavlenko (2002), and Sutton et al. (2007) support this, by describing a person's first language as the language of 'emotional expressiveness', and the second language associated with 'emotional distance'. The more familiar and comfortable that participants were with a language, then the easier it was to access emotions and personal, deeper issues and experiences. These findings reflect other research such as that of Harris et al. (2006) and Sutton et al. (2007) who say that proficiency in a language can impact on the processing of emotional words.

What this study adds to such research, is that at least for some participants (e.g. Cadi and Ffion), the language they described as most familiar and comfortable, was not always their mother-tongue or first language. Ffion described Welsh to be both her mother-tongue and first language, yet due to spending much time speaking English in her early adulthood, she found English easier for accessing emotions and more personal experiences. Cadi also initially described Welsh to be both her mother-tongue and first language. However, after describing her comfort to lie with speaking English, she then changed to describing English as her first language. Dewaele (2009) also describe other cases of bilinguals who prefer to talk about emotion in a non-native language. This highlights not only the changing nature of comfort levels with different languages for these bilinguals, but also suggests that there may be a difference of meaning (for some individuals) between mother-tongue and first language. In terms of the changing nature of which language feels most familiar, there is some relevant literature to be found. Gathercole and Thomas (2009) studied bilingual speakers in Wales. They found that regardless of home language and background, individuals developed equal command of English. The command of Welsh, however, was found to correlate with the level of input of Welsh. This may go some way in explaining the change in ease of using mother-tongue described by Cadi and Ffion – that is, the command of Welsh was decreased due to lack of input of Welsh. But, it does not explain the difficulties that Gwenno and Sian had in speaking English. My findings suggest that Welsh speaking bilinguals may not, in fact, have equal command of the English language where talking about emotions and personal issues are concerned. Further research may be needed in this area.

Another aspect of language described as important by this study, was that of identity and culture. Speaking Welsh has been described by most of the participants as part of who they are, reflecting their culture and identity. Cloke et al. (1997) highlight the important role of the Welsh language in cultural identity for the Welsh, and this is further supported by this study. Furthermore, others such as Coupland and Aldridge (2009), have expanded upon the important role played by the Welsh language within rural Wales. In particular, this has a relevance to the participants in this study who are all from rural Wales. There may be more to be discovered about the role of a rural upbringing within counselling and so there could be potential for further re-search in this area. This aspect also suggests a limitation to the study in that all the participants came from the Gwynedd county of Wales, and it has been said that national identity in Wales varies from region to region (Thompson and Day 1999). The importance of language in identity and culture, and the awareness of this by the therapist, is supported in the literature (e.g. Clauss 1998; Griner and Smith 2006). It may be important particularly for the Welsh as it has been said that the Welsh see their fellow countrymen in an especially favourable light (Bourhis et al. 1973). Although this study suggests a preference for a therapist of similar ethnicity, the literature on this is uncertain (Ramos-Sanchez 2009; Verdinelli and Biever 2013). However, what has been found is that it can be beneficial to therapy when the therapist shows respect, humbleness, curiosity and interest in a client's background and life-experience (Verdinelli and Biever 2013). It may be that these participants feel that without the Welsh language, they cannot be seen in full; that part of who they are is missing from the therapist's view. This aspect can be strongly linked to the feeling that the participants describe of being understood and accepted by their therapist. Gwenno, for example, suggests it can be a barrier to the relationship when it is felt that a therapist does not understand and accept the part that Welsh language and culture plays in who she is as a person. Participants describe a pre-existing bond with other Welsh people that contributes to enhancing their relationship with the Counsellor. Segrott (2001) and Clifford (1997) support this by associating Welsh culture and language as aspects that form strong bonds of belonging and means of connection to others.

Feeling understood and accepted are critical aspects of the therapeutic process (Merry 2002). Rogers (1957) describes the therapeutic relationship, and the delivery and receipt of six core conditions as being at the heart of Person-Centred counselling and therapeutic change. Empathy is described as the Counsellor's ability to enter the client's frame of reference, and unconditional positive regard refers to the Counsellor's non-judgemental acceptance of the client as a person (Merry 2002). Questions have been raised by this study's participants about whether or not they feel understood, or accepted, by a non-Welsh speaking Counsellor. These questions imply that mother-tongue can play a crucial role in the delivery, and more so in the receipt of the core conditions, therefore creating a barrier to therapeutic change. It is important to note, however, that not all of the participants felt that there was a lack of understanding by their therapist. Cadi, for example, felt that she was completely understood by her English speaking therapist, and that her therapist didn't have to be Welsh to understand or see her. It may be important to note that Cadi was the only one who described not being in tune with Welsh culture, describing herself more in tune with English culture. This may suggest that although understanding of Welsh culture was not important to her, it may be that an understanding of her particular culture was. This may be an area for further research. The importance of culture-sensitive therapy has also been described by others (Griner and Smith 2006; Santiago-Rivera 1995). It has been suggested that a person may experience different aspects of the self in different languages, and therefore the existence of dual self or dual identity (e.g. Altarriba 2003; Amati-Mehler et al. 1993; Burck 2004; Perez-Foster 1996; Tehrani and Vaughan 2009). This idea of dual identity may be supported by other descriptions of how different languages come with different emotional and cultural dimensions (Altarriba and Santiago-Rivera 1994; Altarriba and Soltano 1996; de Zulueta 1995). These finding resonate, to some degree, with some of the study's participants, in that they (although not all) describe feeling different when talking Welsh to when talking English. This may further suggest that there are some aspects and emotions that are not accessible in one language, but are in another. For example, Ffion says: *"But then there's that aspect of speaking Welsh where there are certain things that I just can't say in English. It sort of comes from somewhere else almost"* (Ffion). This aspect has been strongly supported by others (e.g. Kokaliari et al. 2013; Marcos and Urcuyo 1979; Santiago-

271

Rivera et al. 2009). The above considers more subtle aspects of language that may influence access to emotions and personal issues, and experiences within counselling. The participants also, however, described more specific aspects of language that impacted on their therapy. Two predominant barriers to therapy, where language is concerned for these participants, were not being able to find the right words, and the aspect of losing the meaning of what they wanted to say. This study highlights, in particular, the gravity of what they mean can be lost, and that this may lead to feeling misunderstood. This work supports research by others (e.g. Damasio 2003; Dewaele 2004, 2008; Iannaco 2009; Imberti 2007; Heredia and Altarriba 2001; LeDoux 1998; Sutton et al. 2007) that highlights the difficulty in translating identical meaning from one language to another, in particular emotional words. Again, as described above, feeling understood is a crucial aspect of effective counselling (Merry 2002). Therefore, it will be important for the Counsellor to be aware that a word may not hold the same meaning in English as it does in Welsh.

With further relevance to counselling, this study describes how difficulties finding words and expressing meaning can result in changing the felt feeling, for example, to one of *"frustration"* (Gwenno) or *"confusion"* (Sian). Such interference may be problematic to the therapeutic process, preventing the development of insights and understanding, by not accommodating sticking with feelings as they arise – a process considered important in Person-Centred Counselling (Mearns and Thorne 2013). On the other hand, it may be also worth noting that these feelings elicited by language difficulties, that have been described by the participants, can in themselves open a whole new area of personal discovery, and that this may be beneficial to the client. Gwenno, for example, described feeling less confident in speaking English (her second language) – a feeling also described by others in the literature (Segalowitz 1976). Although this was described as a negative aspect of therapy, it was also described as positive, as it allowed her to identify this lack of confidence and explore it further, strengthening her relationship with her therapist. This phenomenon has also been described by Costa (2010). Hidden areas of personal issues have been described in the cases of all participants in this current study. This may be a useful insight for the Counsellor working with Welsh clients, that is, there may be more to the struggle of searching for words than meets the eye. An example of this might be the cases of Cadi and Ffion. It has been said that speaking in a second language 'challenges early attachment relationships to the primary language and may lead to unconscious internal conflicts about ties to the past and the present' (Kokaliari et al. 2013, p. 99). Some such conflicts were described by Ffion and Cadi, and, without considering the role of language in therapy, such issues that may be of great importance for personal development may have been overlooked. Aspects important to developing a trusting and facilitative relationship with the Counsellor have been described above, in particular, with regards to feeling understood and accepted, and the inherent role of culture and identity. Another important role of language in the therapeutic relationship is that of safety. All participants described language as a way of offering safety within the counselling relationship. For those who described Welsh as their first language, speaking Welsh, and having a Welsh therapist, felt safer. For Cadi, English was safer, but what is important is that language (regardless of which language) was an important aspect of safety. As safety is a crucial aspect of counselling (Mearns and Thorne 2013; Proctor 2002), it will be important for Counsellors working with Welsh speaking clients to consider this aspect in their work together.

Finally, the study also described 'extras' that language brought into the counselling context, in particular bilingualism. For example, because a person had access to more than one language, it was considered to give more flexibility within counselling. The first flexibility described was that of choice; being bilingual meant you could choose the language in which to undergo counselling. Having a choice was felt important by the participants. However, when the choice was limited, or taken away, as it was for Gwenno, this contributed to a negative experience of counselling. Furthermore, it was considered that having two languages felt like there were more options within the therapy, in the sense that an individual could switch from one language to the other depending on what felt easier at the time, or depending on how much distance they might want to put between them and the subject. For example: *"So, if I'm trying to distance myself somehow, for whatever reasons, erm ... then sometimes it's easier to do that in English compared to Welsh. So really, when I'm trying to get really close to something, I find it easier doing that in Welsh"* (Sian). This aspect relates to research by Sutton et al. (2007) that describes second language as the language of 'emotional distance'. This switching from one language to another has been described by others (e.g. Kokaliari et al. 2013; Bowker and Richards 2004). Another benefit of switching between languages that has been described, is that of strengthening the bond between client and therapist (Santiago-Rivera et al. 2009). This benefit was described also in this study by Ffion. However, it may be important to note that this positive aspect of therapy for bilinguals may be missing for some, such as Gwenno, where their therapists do not speak both languages. This difficulty has also been described from the perspective of the therapist and may be an area for further study (Verdinelli and Biever 2009).

Conclusion

Although the inclusion criteria allowed for variability in both gender and experience, the sample did not include any male participants, nor any non-Counsellor or trainee Counsellor participants. I originally felt that it would be important to include such participants as it was my belief that trainee Counsellors or Counsellors have been given the opportunity to develop their ability in talking about emotions and feelings to a greater level than other individuals in the population might. In particular, here, Welsh speaking trainee Counsellors or Counsellors will have had to do this through their second language (English) due to the lack of Counselling courses that are taught through the Welsh language. For this reason, their experience of talking about emotional issues may be different to others who may not be as comfortable talking English, or even about feelings. What I found, however, was that although participants agreed that there were others in Wales who were less confident in Welsh, within the sample itself, I discovered various degrees of comfort, and this turned out to be an interesting aspect of the findings. Another limitation to consider may be the use of IPA. Although there are many benefits of IPA (Smith et al. 2009), there are also limitations that need to be recognized (Smith et al. 2009; Willig 2008). One limitation is its dependency on language as its main tool of access. Although there is no room here to do this justice (Willig 2008), it may be important to keep a close eye on this limitation, in particular in this study, due to the importance of language in the topic matter. In light of the findings, and particularly with reference to those describing difficulties that first language speakers have in expressing themselves in English, I recognize that an obvious limitation to this study is that the interviews themselves were conducted in English. Due to the difficulties described by Sian and Gwenno in particular, it may be that due to the interviews being conducted in English, this particular study may not have had access to some experiences. The reason, however, why I chose to interview in English, as opposed to interviewing in Welsh and then translating the data into English for presentation, is that the process of translating would increase the likelihood of meaning loss and because there are not always direct translations (Iannaco 2009; Sutton et al. 2007). However, the participants checking their own translated transcripts (member checks) ensured validity and picked up any loss of meaning or misinterpretation. Furthermore it is important to note that meaningful knowledge has been obtained in similar situations by conducting interviews in English (Costa 2010). There may be some aspects of Welsh mother-tongue individuals' experiences that cannot be accessed through the English language, and some meaning may have been lost. I would like to believe that through using member checks, being Welsh myself, and being aware of the issue, that these limitations have been minimized. However, it may be relevant to conduct such studies about the importance of Welsh in the counselling context and the counselling relationship through the medium of Welsh.

It appears that for this study's participants, mother-tongue is important in accessing emotional and personal experiences, and an important aspect of their identity and culture. They have described that it can be a barrier to therapeutic change when absent (e.g. loss of meaning and words), and to creating a trusting relationship with the Counsellor (e.g. not feeling safe or understood). It has also been described as benefiting counselling by providing flexibility and a deeper connection with their emotions, and therapist, when present. The participants in this study have also shown that issues around mother-tongue can be important in addressing hidden issues that may be crucial for personal development. The results suggest that it will be important for the Counsellor to consider a client's language, what it means to them, and how it might impact the material that is covered, as well as the relationship. Although it does not suggest that no therapeutic benefit is possible when clients are not able to speak their mother-tongue, it does suggest (as does the literature) that it is important that they demonstrate interest and sensitivity in the client's language, and in the struggle and difficulties that arise when they are not able to communicate using their mother-tongue. The results of this study provides further support to the importance of mother-tongue in therapy and in the counselling relationship. However, it highlights the individual nature of this importance. The case of Cadi, in particular, in this study, goes far in suggesting caution with a one size fits all approach to the role of language in Counselling.

REFERENCES

Adams, R.G., & Blieszner, R. (1994). An integrative conceptual framework for friendship research. *Journal of Social and Personal Relationships,* 11(2): 163–184.

Adewuya, A.O., Ologun, Y.A., & Ibigbami, O.S. (2006). Post-traumatic stress disorder after childbirth in Nigerian women: Prevalence and risk factors. *BJOG: An International Journal of Obstetrics and Gynaecology,* 113: 284–288.

Agnew-Davies, R. (1999). Learning from research into the counselling relationship. In C. Feltham (Ed.). *Understanding the Counselling Relationship.* London, UK: Sage Publications.

Ainsworth, M.S. (1991). Attachments and other affectional bonds across the life cycle. In C.M. Parkes, J. Stevenson-Hinds, & P. Marris (Eds.). *Attachment Across the Lifecycle.* New York, NY: Routledge.

Albin, D.D. (2006). Making the boy (w)hole: A semiotic exploration of body modifications. *Psychodynamic Practice,* 12(1): 19–35.

Alcina, M. (2009). *Tattoos as personal narrative.* (Unpublished Doctoral thesis: University of New Orleans).

Alcorn, K.L., O'Donovan, A., Patrick, J.C., Creedy, D., & Devilly, G.J. (2010). A prospective longitudinal study of the prevalence of post-traumatic stress disorder resulting from childbirth events. *Psychological Medicine,* 40: 1849–1859.

Alhanati, B.S. (2007). *How does becoming and being a professional counsellor affect one's personal life? A qualitative exploration.* (Unpublished Master's thesis: University of Victoria, Canada).

Allan, G., & Adams, R.G. (1989). Ageing and the structure of friendship, in R.G. Adams & R. Blieszner (Eds.). *Older Adult Friendship.* Newbury Park, CA: Sage Publications.

Allen, K. (1995). Coping with life changes and transitions: The role of pets. *Interactions,* 13(3): 5–8.

Allen, S. (1998). A qualitative analysis of the process, mediating variables and the impact of traumatic childbirth. *Journal of Reproductive and Infant Psychology,* 16: 107–131.

References

Altarriba, J. (2003). Does caring equal liking? A theoretical approach to conceptual non-equivalence between languages. *International Journal of Bilingualism*, 7(3): 305–322.

Altarriba, J., Bauer, L.M., & Benvenuto, C. (1999). Concreteness, context-availability, and imageability ratings and word associations for abstract, concrete, and emotion words. *Behavior Research Methods, Instruments, & Computers*, 31(4): 578–602.

Altarriba, J., & Santiago-Rivera, A. (1994). Current perspectives on using linguistic and cultural factors in counselling the Hispanic client. *Professional Psychology Research and Practice*, 25(4): 388–397.

Altarriba, J., & Soltano, E. (1996). Repetition blindness and bilingual memory, token individuation for translation equivalents. *Memory and Cognition*, 24(6): 700–711.

Amati-Mehler, J., Argentieri, S., & Canestri, J. (1993). *The Babel of the Unconscious: Mother tongue and foreign languages in the psychoanalytical dimension.* Madison, CT: International Universities Press.

American Psychiatric Association (1980). *Diagnostic and Statistical Manual of Mental Disorders* (3rd Edition). Washington, DC: American Psychiatric Association.

American Psychiatric Association (1994). *Diagnostic and Statistical Manual of Mental Disorders* (4th Edition). Washington, DC: American Psychiatric Association.

Anastasia, D.J.M. (2009). Living marked: Tattooed women, embodiment, and identity. *Humanities and Social Sciences*, 69(9-A): 3759.

Anderson, B. (1983). *Imagined Communities.* London, UK: Verso.

Anderson, C.A., and Hammen, C.L. (1993). Psychosocial outcomes of children of unipolar depressed, bipolar, medically ill, and normal women: A longitudinal study. *Journal of Consulting and Clinical Psychology*, 61: 448–454.

Anderson, R.K., Hart, B.L., & Hart, L.A. (Eds.). (1984). *The Pet Connection: Its influence on our health and quality of life.* Minneapolis, MN: University of Minnesota.

Anooshian, L.J., & Hertel, P.T. (1994). Emotionality in free recall: Language specificity in bilingual memory. *Cognition and Emotion*, 8(6): 503–514.

Aponte, H.J., & Winter, J.E. (2013). The person and practice of the therapist. In M. Baldwin (Ed.). *The Use of Self in Therapy*. Hove, UK: Routledge.

Archer, J. (1999). *The Nature of Grief: The evolution and psychology of reactions to loss*. London, UK: Routledge.

Aristotle (1990). In A.W. Price. (Ed.). *Love and Friendship in Plato and Aristotle*. London, UK: Clarendon Paperbacks.

Armstrong, M. (1994). Tattoos: A risk-taking art, *Texas Nursing*, 63: 8–9.

Atkinson, M. (2002). Pretty in ink: Conformity, resistance, and negotiation in women's tattooing, *Sex Roles*, 47, (5/6): 232.

Atkinson, M. (2004). Tattooing and civilizing processes: Body modification as self-control. *The Canadian Review of Sociology and Anthropology*, 41: 125–147.

Ayers, S. (2004). Delivery as a traumatic event: Prevalence, risk factors, screening and treatment. *Clinical Obstetrics and Gynaecology*, 47(3): 552–567.

Ayers, S. (2007). Thoughts and emotions during traumatic birth: A qualitative study. *Birth*, 34: 3.

Ayers, S., Eagle, A., & Waring, H. (2006). The effects of childbirth-related post-traumatic stress disorder on women and their relationships: A qualitative study. *Psychology, Health and Medicine*, 11: 389–398.

Ayers, S., Harris, R., Sawyer, A., Parfitt, Y., & Ford, E. (2009). Posttraumatic stress disorder after childbirth: Analysis of symptom presentation and sampling. *Journal of Affective Disorders*, 119: 200–204.

Ayers, S., McKenzie-McHarg, K., & Eagle, A. (2007a). Cognitive behavioural therapy for post-traumatic stress disorder: Case studies. *Journal of Psychosomatic Obstetrics and Gynaecology*, 28(3): 177–184.

References

Ayers, S., Wright, D.B., & Wells, N. (2007b). Symptoms of post-traumatic stress disorder in couples after birth: Association with the couple's relationship and parent-baby bond. *Journal of Reproductive and Infant Psychology*, 25(1): 40–50.

BACP (2013). *BACP Ethical Framework for Good Practice in Counselling and Psychotherapy*. Lutterworth, UK: British Association for Counselling and Psychotherapy.

Bailham, D., & Joseph, S., (2003). Post-traumatic stress following childbirth: A review of the emerging literature and directions for research and practice. *Psychology, Health and Medicine*, 8: 159–168.

Baldwin, M. (3rd Edition) (2013). Interview with Carl Rogers on the use of self in therapy. In M. Baldwin (Ed.). *The Use of Self in Therapy*. Hove, UK: Routledge.

Ballard, C.G., Stanley A.K., & Brockington I.F. (1995). Post-traumatic stress disorder after childbirth. *British Journal of Psychiatry*, 166: 525–528.

Bancroft, L. (2002). *Why Does He Do That? Inside the minds of angry and controlling men*. New York, NY: Berkley Books.

Banning, N. (2012). When the therapist is a horse. *Therapy Today*, 23(2): 14–18.

Barlow, C.A., & Phelan, A.M. (2007). Peer collaboration: A model to support counsellor self-care. *Canadian Journal of Counselling*, 41(1): 3–15.

Barnett, M. (2007). What brings you here? An exploration of the unconscious motivations of those who choose to train and work as psychotherapists and counsellors. *Psychodynamic Practice*, 13(3): 257–274.

Beck, A.M., & Katcher, A.H. (1996). *Between Pets and People. The importance of animal companionship*. (Revised Edition). West Lafayette, IN: Purdue University Press.

Beck, A.M., & Katcher, A.H. (2003). Future directions in human–animal bond research. *American Behavior Scientist*, 47(1): 79–93.

Beck, C.T. (1999). Postpartum depression: Stopping the thief that steals motherhood. *AWHONN Lifelines*, 3: 41–44.

Beck, C.T. (2004a). Birth trauma: In the eye of the beholder. *Nursing Research*, 53: 28–35.

Beck, C.T. (2004b). Post-traumatic stress disorder due to childbirth: The aftermath. *Nursing Research*, 53: 216–224.

Beck, C.T., & Watson, S. (2010). Subsequent childbirth after a previous traumatic birth. *Nursing Research*, 59, (4): 241–249.

Beck, C.T. & Watson, S.D. (2008). Impact of birth trauma on breastfeeding: A tale of two pathways. *Nursing Research*, 57(4): 228–236.

Becker, M.E. (1998). The abuse excuse and patriarchal narratives. *Northwestern University Law Review*, 92(4): 1459–1480.

Becvar, D.S. (2003). The impact on the family therapist of a focus on death, dying and bereavement. *Journal of Marital and Family Therapy*, 29(4): 469–477.

Beder, J. (2004). Lessons about bereavement. *Journal of Loss and Trauma*, 9: 383–387.

Birth Trauma Association (n.d.), retrieved January 10, 2014, from http://www.birthtraumaassociation.org.uk/

Blue, G.F. (1986). The value of pets in children's lives. *Childhood Education*, 63(2): 84–90.

Boelen, P.A., van de Schoot, R., van den Hout, M.A., de Keijser, J., & van den Bout, J. (2010). Prolonged grief disorder, depression, and posttraumatic stress disorder are distinguishable syndromes. *Journal of Affective Disorders*, 125: 374–378.

Boelan, P.A., & van den Bout, J. (2008). Complicated grief and uncomplicated grief are distinguishable constructs. *Psychiatry Research*, 157: 311–314.

Bonanno, G.A. (2009). *The Other Side of Sadness*. New York, NY: Basic Books.

Bonanno, G.A., & Keltner, D. (2004). The coherence of emotion systems: Comparing on-line measures of appraisal and facial expressions, and self-report. *Cognition & Emotion*, 18: 431–444.

Bonanno, G.A., Neria, Y., Mancini, A., Coifman, K., Litz, B., & Insel, B. (2007). Is there more to complicated grief than depression and posttraumatic stress disorder? A test of incremental validity. *Journal of Abnormal Psychology*, 116(2): 342–351.

References

Bourhis, R.Y., Giles, H., & Tajfel, H. (1973). Language as a determinant of Welsh identity. *European Journal of Social Psychology*, 3(4): 447–460.

Bowker, P., & Richards, B. (2004). Speaking the same language? A qualitative study of therapists' experiences of working in English with proficient bilingual clients. *Psychodynamic Practice*, 10(4): 459–478.

Bowlby, J. (1973). *Attachment and Loss. Vol. 2: Separation: Anxiety and anger*. New York, NY: Basic Books.

Bowlby, J. (1980). *Attachment and Loss. Vol. 3: Loss: Sadness and depression*. New York, NY: Basic Books.

Bradshaw, J. (2011). *In Defence of Dogs*. London, UK: Penguin Books Ltd.

Bradshaw, J. (2013). *Cat Sense: The feline enigma revealed*. London, UK: Penguin Books Ltd.

Brady, J.L., Healy, F.C., Norcross, J.C., & Guy, J.D. (1995). Stress in counsellors: An integrative research review. In W. Dryden (Ed.). *The Stresses of Counselling in Action*. London, UK: Sage Publications.

Brown, B.B. (1981). A life-span approach to friendship: Age-related dimensions of an ageless relationship. *Research in the Interweave of Social Roles*, (2): 23–50.

Brown, L.S. (1995). Not outside the range: One feminist perspective on trauma. In C. Caruth (Ed.). *Trauma Explorations in Memory*. Baltimore, MD: Johns Hopkins University Press.

Browning, D. (2003). Pathos, paradox and poetics: Grounded theory and the experience of bereavement. *Smith College Studies in Social Work*, 73(3): 325–336.

Bruner, J. (1990). *Acts of Meaning*. Cambridge, MA: Harvard University Press.

Bryant-Jefferies, R. (2006). *Counselling for Death and Dying: Person-centred dialogues*. Abingdon, UK: Radcliffe Publishing Ltd.

Buchanan, L., & Hughes, R. (2000). *Experiences of Person-Centred Counsellor Training*. Ross-on-Wye, UK: PCCS Books.

Bukowski, W.M., & Hoza, B. (1989). Popularity and friendship: Issues in theory, measurement and outcome. In T.J. Berndt &

G.W. Ladd. (Eds.). *Peer Relationships in Child Development*. New York, NY: John Wiley & Sons.

Burck, C. (1997). Language and narrative: Learning from bilingualism. In R.K. Papadopoulos, & J. Byng-Hall (Eds.). *Multiple Voices: Narrative in systemic family psychotherapy* (2nd Edition). London, UK: Duckworth.

Burck, C. (2004). Living in several languages: Implications for therapy. *Journal of Family Therapy*, 26(4): 314–339.

Buxbaum, E. (1949). The role of a second language in the formation of Ego and Superego. *Psychoanalytic Quarterly*, 18: 279–289.

Calhoun, L.G., & Tedeschi, R.G. (1998). Posttraumatic growth: Future directions. In R.G. Tedeshci, C.L. Park, & L.G. Calhoun (Eds.). *Posttraumatic growth: Positive changes in the aftermath of crisis*. Mahwah, NJ: Lawrence Erlbaum Associates, Publishers.

Calhoun, L.G., & Tedeschi, R.G. (2000). Posttraumatic growth: The positive lessons of loss. In R. Neimeyer (Ed.). *Meaning Reconstruction and the Experience of Loss*. Washington, DC: American Psychological Association.

Campbell, C.I., & Alexander, J.A. (2002). Culturally competent treatment practices and ancillary service use in outpatient substance abuse treatment. *Journal of Substance Abuse Treatment*, 22: 109–119.

Carll, E.K. (Ed.). (2007). *Trauma Psychology: Issues in violence, disaster, health, and illness*. Westport, CT: Praeger.

Carlyle, K.E., Slater, M.D., & Chakroff, J.L. (2008). Newspaper coverage of intimate partner violence: Skewing representations of risk. *Journal of Communication*, 58: 168–186.

Carroll, M. (1996). *Counselling Supervision Theory, Skills and Practice*. London, UK: Sage Publications.

Caruth, C. (1996). *Unclaimed Experience: Trauma, narrative and history*. Baltimore, MD: The Johns Hopkins University Press.

Casemore, R. (2006). *Person-Centred Counselling in a Nutshell*. London, UK: Sage Publications.

Cavanaugh, L.A., Leonard, H.A., & Scammon, D.L. (2008). A tale of two personalities: How canine companions shape relationships and well-being. *Journal of Business Research*. 61: 469–479.

References

Cawkhill, P. (2002). Does counselling damage your relationship? *Counselling and Psychotherapy Journal*, 13(4), 41–42.

Chur-Hansen, A., Winefield, H.R., & Beckwith, M. (2009). Companion animals for elderly women: The importance of attachment. *Qualitative Research in Psychology*, 6(4): 281–293.

Clauss, C.S. (1998). Language: The unspoken variable in psychotherapy practice. *Psychotherapy*, 35(2): 188–196.

Clifford, J. (1997). *Routes: Travel and translation in the late twentieth century.* Cambridge, MA: Harvard University Press.

Cloke, P., Goodwin, M., & Milbourne, P. (1997). *Rural Wales. Community and Marginalization.* Cardiff, UK: University of Wales Press.

Cogan, T. (1977). *A Study of Friendship Among Psychotherapists.* (Unpublished Doctoral thesis: University of Illinois, IL).

Cogill, S.R., Caplan, H.L., Alexandra, H., Robson, K.M., & Kumar, R. (1986). Impact of maternal postnatal depression on cognitive development of young children. *British Medical Journal*, 292: 1165–1167.

Collins, K.A. (2008). *A qualitative exploration of the impact of personal development in counselling training on the student counsellors' significant relationships: Should counsellor training come with a stronger warning or more support?* (Unpublished MA dissertation: University of Chester, UK).

Comas-Diaz, L., & Jacobsen, F. (1991). Ethnocultural transference and countertransference in the therapeutic dyad. *American Journal of Orthopsychiatry*, 61(3): 392–402.

Comas-Diaz, L., & Weiner, M.B. (2013). Sisters of the heart: How women's friendships heal. *Women and Therapy*, 36(1–2): 1–10.

Connor, M. (1994). *Training the Counsellor: An integrative model.* London, UK: Routledge.

Cooper, M. (2008). *Essential Research Findings in Counselling and Psychotherapy: The facts are friendly.* London, UK: Sage Publications.

Coren, S. (2012). Canine Empathy: Your dog really does care if you are unhappy. *Psychology Today. Canine Corner.* Retrieved from http://www.psychology today.com.

Corson, S.A., & Corson, E. (1980). Pet animals as nonverbal communication mediators in psychotherapy in institutional settings. In S.A. Corson, & E. Corson (Eds.). *Ethology and Nonverbal Communication in Mental Health*. Oxford: Pergamon Press.

Costa, B. (2010). Mother-tongue or non-native language? Learning from conversations with bilingual/multilingual therapists about working with clients who do not share their native language. *Ethnicity and Inequalities in Health and Social Care*, 3(1): 15–24.

Coupland, N., & Aldridge, M., (2009). Introduction: A critical approach to the revitalisation of Welsh. *International Journal of the Sociology of Language*, 195: 5–13.

Cowan, R. (2012). Lasting the course. *Therapy Today*, July: 14–17.

Cramer, D. (1994). Self-esteem and Rogers' core conditions in close friends: A latent variable path analysis of panel data. *Counselling Psychology Quarterly*, 7(3): 327–337.

Cranton, P. (1997). *Transformative Learning in Action: Insights from practice*. San Francisco, CA: Jossey Bass.

Creedy, D.K., Shochet, I.M., & Horsfall, J. (2000). Childbirth and the development of acute trauma symptoms: Incidence and contributing factors. *Birth*, 27: 104–111.

Cusack, O. (1988). *Pets and Mental Health*. New York, NY: Haworth.

Cusack, O., & Smith, E. (1984). *Pets and the Elderly: The therapeutic bond*. New York, NY: Haworth.

Custance, D., & Mayer, J. (2012). Empathic-like responding by domestic dogs (Canis familiaris) to distress in humans: An exploratory study, *Animal Cognition*, 15: 851–859.

Cutcliffe, J.R. (1998). Hope, counselling and complicated grief reactions. *Journal of Advanced Nursing*, 28(4): 754–761.

Damasio, A. (2003). *Looking for Spinosa: Joy, sorrow and the feeling brain*. London, UK: Heinemann.

Davies, E. (2011) (IAITH: Welsh Centre for Language Planning for the Department for Health, Social Services and Children, Welsh Government and the Care Council for Wales). Welsh speakers' experiences of Health and Social Care services. *Welsh*

References

Assembly Government (http://www.iaith.eu/uploads/welsh_speakers_experiences_of_health_and_social_care.pdf) Accessed January, 9, 2013.

DeHart, D.D., Follingstad, D.R., & Fields, A.M. (2010). Does context matter in determining psychological abuse? Effects of pattern, harm, relationship, and norms. *Journal of Family Violence*, 25: 461–474.

DeMello, M. (2000). *Bodies of Inscription: A cultural history of the modern tattoo community.* Durham, NC: Duke University Press.

Demir, M., & Weitenkamp, L. (2007). "I am so happy because today I have found my friend": Friendship and personality as predictors of happiness. *Journal of Happiness Studies*, 8(2): 181–211.

Denscombe, M. (2014). *The Good Research Guide. For small-scale social research projects* (5th Edition). Maidenhead, UK: Open University Press.

Denzin, N., & Lincoln, Y. (Eds.). (2005). *The Sage Handbook of Qualitative Research.* London, UK: Sage Publications.

Deutsch, C.J. (1984). Self-reported sources of stress among psychotherapists. *Professional Psychology: Research and Practice*, 15: 833–845.

Dewaele, J. (2009). Age effects on self-perceived communicative competence and language choice among adult multi-linguals. *EUROSLA Yearbook*, 9 (1): 245–268.

Dewaele, J.M. (2004). The emotional force of swear words and taboo words in the speech of multilinguals. *Journal of Multicultural and Multilingual Development*, 25(2–3): 204–222.

Dewaele, J.M. (2008). The emotional weight of 'I love you' in multilinguals' languages. *Journal of Pragmatics*, 40: 1753–1780.

Dewaele, J.M., & Pavlenko, A. (2002). Emotion vocabulary in interlanguage. *Language Learning*, 52(2): 263–322.

Dexter, G.L. (1996). *A critical review of the impact of counselling training courses on trainees.* (Unpublished Doctoral thesis: University of Durham, UK).

de Zulueta, F. (1990). Bilingualism and family therapy. *Journal of Family Therapy*, 12: 255–265.

de Zulueta, F. (1995). Bilingualism, culture and identity. *Group Analysis*, 28(2): 179–190.

Dirkx J.M. (2001). Transformative learning and the power of individuation. *ERIC Digest*: 223.

Donati, M., & Watts, M. (2005). Personal development in counsellor training: Towards clarification of inter-related concepts. *British Journal of Guidance and Counselling*, 33(4): 475–484.

Dubinsky, A., & Bazhenova, O. (1997). 'Moments of discovery, times of learning', In S. Reid (Ed). *Developments in Infant Observation: The Tavistock Model*. London, UK: Routledge.

Dueckman, A. (2012). Killing her softly. *Canadian Mennonite*, 16(14): 4–7.

Dunphy, R., & Schniering, C.A. (2009). The experience of counselling the bereaved. *The Humanistic Psychologist*, 37: 353–369.

Dutton, D.G., & Painter, S. (1993). The Battered Woman Syndrome: Effects of severity and intermittency of abuse. *American Journal of Orthopsychiatry*, 63: 614–621.

Dryden, W. (2008). The therapeutic alliance as an integrating framework. In W. Dryden (Ed.). *Key Issues for Counselling in Action* (2nd Edition). London, UK: Sage Publications.

Dryden, W. & Thorne, B. (1991). *Training and Supervision for Counselling in Action*. London, UK: Sage Publications.

Egan, G. (1973). *Face to Face*. Monterey, CA: Brooks/Cole.

Elmir, R., Schmied, V., Wilkes, L., & Jackson, D. (2010). Women's perceptions and experiences of a traumatic birth: A meta-ethnography. *Journal of Advanced Nursing*, 66(10): 2142–2153.

Elmir, R., Schmied, V., Wilkes, L., & Jackson, D. (2011). Separation, failure and temporary relinquishment: Women's experiences of early mothering in the context of emergency hysterectomy. *Journal of Clinical Nursing*, 21: 1119–1127.

Engel, B. (2002). *The Emotionally Abusive Relationship: How to stop being abused and how to stop abusing*. Hoboken, NJ: John Wiley & Sons.

Erikson, E. (1993). *Childhood and Society*. New York, NY: Norton.

References

Ervin, S. (1964). Language and TAT content in bilinguals. *Journal of Abnormal and Social Psychology*, 63: 500–507.

Etherington, K. (2003). *Trauma, the body and transformation*. London, UK: Jessica Kingsley Publications.

Etherington, K. (2004). *Becoming a Reflective Researcher: Using our selves in research*. London, UK: Jessica Kingsley Publishers.

Eubanks, V. (1996). Zones of Dither: Writing the postmodern body. *Body and Society*, 2(3): 73–88.

Evans, P. (1993). *Verbal Abuse Survivors Speak Out: On relationship and Recovery*. Avon Massachusetts: Adams Media Corporation.

Evans, P. (2000). *The Verbally Abusive Relationship: How to recognise it and how to respond* (3rd Ed.). Avon, MA: Adams Media Corporation.

Farber, B.A. (1983). The effects of psychotherapeutic practice on psychotherapists. *Psychotherapy: Theory, research and practice*, 20: 2.

Farber, B.A., Manevich, I., Metzger, J., & Saypol, S. (2005). Choosing psychotherapy as a career: Why did we cross that road? *Journal of Clinical Psychology*, 61(8): 1009–1031.

Farber, B.A., & Norcross, J.C. (2005). Choosing psychotherapy as a career: Beyond "Why do we want to help people". *Journal of Clinical Psychology*, 61(8): 939–943.

Favali, V., & Milton, M. (2010). Disabled horse-riders' experience of horse-riding: A phenomenological analysis of the benefits of contact with animals. *Existential Analysis,* 21(2): 251–262.

Fawcett, N.R., & Gullone, G. (2001). Cute and cuddly and a whole lot more? A call for empirical investigation into therapeutic benefits of Human–animal Interaction for children. *Behaviour Change*, 18(2): 124–133.

Fear, R. (2004). One training voice: Reflecting on the echoes. In V. Harding-Davies, G. Alred, K. Hunt, & G. Davies (Eds.). *Experiences of Counsellor Training: Challenge, surprise and change*. Basingstoke, UK: Palgrave MacMillan.

FEDIAF. The European Pet Food Industry Federation (2012). *Facts and Figures 2012*. Retrieved from http://www.fediaf.org/facts-figures/

Field, N.P., & Filanosky, C. (2010). Continuing bonds, risk factors for complicated grief and adjustment to bereavement. *Death Studies*, 34: 1–29.

Field, T., Healy, B., Goldstein, S., & Guthertz, M. (1990). Behaviour state matching and synchrony in mother-infant interaction of non-depressed versus depressed dyads. *Developmental Psychology*, 26: 7–14.

Finlay, L. (2008). A dance between the reduction and reflexivity: Explicating the phenomenological psychological attitude, *Journal of Phenomenological Psychology*, 39: 1–32.

Fisher, B.S., & Regan, S.L. (2006). The extent and frequency of abuse in the lives of older women and their relationship with health outcomes. *The Gerontologist*, 46(2): 200–209.

Fisher, J.A. (2002). Tattooing the body, marking culture, *Body & Society*, 8(4): 91–107.

Flick, U. (2011). *Introducing Research Methodology*. London, UK: Sage Publications.

Fogle, B. (1983). How did we find our way here? In A.H. Katcher & A. Beck (Eds.). *New Perspectives on our Lives with Companion Animals*. Philadelphia, PA: University of Pennsylvania Press.

Fogle, B. (Ed.). (1981). *Interrelations between People and Pets*. Springfield, IL: Charles C. Thomas.

Follett, J.A. (2009). *The consumption of tattoos and tattooing: The body as permanent text*. (Unpublished Doctoral thesis: University of Wolverhampton, UK).

Follingstad, D.R. (2007). Rethinking current approaches to psychological abuse: Conceptual and methodological issues, *Aggression and Violent Behaviour*, 12(4): 439–458.

Follingstad, D.R. (2011). A measure of severe psychological abuse normed on a nationally representative sample of adults. *Journal of Interpersonal Violence*, 26(6): 1194–1214.

Follingstad, D.R., & DeHart, D.D. (2000). Defining psychological abuse of husbands towards wives: Contexts, behaviours and typologies. *Journal of Interpersonal Violence*, 15(9): 461–474.

Fones, C. (1996). Posttraumatic stress disorder occurring after painful childbirth. *Journal of Nervous and Mental Disease,* 184: 195–196.

Ford, J.D., Tennen, H., & Albert, D. (2008). A contrarian view of growth following adversity. In S. Joseph & P.A. Linley (Eds.). *Trauma, Recovery & Growth: Positive psychological perspectives on posttraumatic stress.* Hoboken, NJ: John Wiley & Sons.

Fox, J., & Jones, K.D. (2013). DSM-5 and bereavement: The loss of normal grief? *Journal of Counseling and Development,* 91(1): 113–119.

Franklin, A. (1999). *Animals and Modern Culture.* London, UK: Sage Publications.

Freud, S. (1917). Mourning and melancholia. In S. Freud (Ed.). *The Standard Edition of the Complete Psychological Works of Sigmund Freud, Volume XIV.* London, UK: Hogarth Press.

Freudenberger, H.J., & Robbins, A. (1979). The hazards of being a psychoanalyst, *The Psychoanalytic Review,* 66: 275–296.

Friedman, E., Katcher, A.H., Lynch, J.J., & Thomas, S.A. (1980). Animal companions and one year survival from coronary care unit. *Public Health Reports,* 95(4): 307–312.

Friedman, J. (1994). *Cultural Identity and Global Processes.* London, UK: Sage Publications.

Gathercole, V.C.M., & Thomas, E.M. (2009). Bilingual first language development: Dominant language takeover, threatened minority language take-up. *Bilingualism Language and Cognition,* 12(2): 213–237.

Gaudio, C.P. (1998). Personal growth of the therapist: Living with loss. *Journal of Family Psychology,* 9(4): 13–31.

Gavin, N.I., Gaynes, B.N., Lohr, K.N., Meltzer-Brody, S., Gartlehner, G., & Swinson, T. (2005). Perinatal depression: A systematic review of prevalence and incidence. *Obstetrics and Gynecology,* 106: 1071–1083.

Gebauer, J.E., Haddock, G., Broemer, P., & von Hecker, U. (2013). The role of semantic self-perceptions in temporal distance perceptions toward autobiographical events: The semantic congruence model. *Journal of Personality and Social Psychology*, 105(5): 852–872.

Geller, E.S. (1982). *Preserving the Environment: New strategies for behaviour change*. Oxford, UK: Pergamon Press.

Gergen, K.J. (1995). Postmodernism as a humanism. *The Humanistic Psychologist*, 23: 71–82.

Getsinger, S.H. (1978). Psychotherapy and the fourth dimension. *Psychotherapy: Theory, research and practice*, 15(3): 216–225.

Giddens, A. (1991). *Modernity and Self-Identity: Self and society in the late modern age*, Cambridge, MA: Blackwell Publishing Ltd.

Gilbert, P. (2005). *Compassion-Conceptualisations, Research and Use in Psychotherapy*. London, UK: Routledge.

Gilbey, A., McNicholas, J., & Collis, G.M. (2007). A longitudinal test of belief that companion animal ownership can help reduce loneliness. *Anthrozos*, 20(4): 345–353.

Giles, H., Taylor, D.M, & Bourhis, R.Y. (1974). Dimensions of Welsh identity. *European Journal of Social Psychology*, 7(2): 165–174.

Gilligan, C. (1996). Centrality of relationship in human development: A puzzle, some evidence, and a theory. In G. Noam & K. Fisher (Eds.). *Development and Vulnerability in Close Relationships*. Mahwah, NJ: Lawrence Erlbaum.

Gladding, S.T. (2004). *Counselling: A comprehensive perspective*. Upper Saddle River, NJ: Merrill/Prentice Hall.

Gockel, A. (2009). Spirituality and the process of healing: A narrative study, *International Journal for the Psychology of Religion*, 19: 217–230.

Goldberg, C. (1986). *On Being a Psychotherapist: The journey of the healer*. New York, NY: Gardner Press.

Golden, A.-M.J., & Dalgleish, T. (2012). Facets of pejorative self-processing in complicated grief. *Journal of Consulting and Clinical Psychology*, 80(3): 512–524.

Goncalves, O.F., & Machado, P.P.P. (2000). Emotions, narrative and change. *European Journal of Psychotherapy, Counselling and Health*, 3(3): 349–360.

Goode, E., & Vail, D.A. (2008). *Extreme Deviance*. London, UK: Sage Publications.

References

Gort, G. (1984). Pathological grief: Causes, recognition, and treatment. *Canadian Family Physician,* 30: 914–924.

Granfanaki, S. (2001). What counselling research has taught us about the concept of congruence: Main discoveries and unresolved issues. In G. Wyatt (Ed.). *Rogers' Therapeutic Conditions: Evolution, theory and practice: Vol. 1. Congruence.* Ross-on-Wye: UK: PCCS Books.

Green, J. (2010). *Creating the Therapeutic Relationship in Counselling and Psychotherapy.* Exeter, UK: Learning Matters.

Greenberg, L.S., & Geller, S.M. (2001). Congruence and therapeutic presence. In G. Wyatt (Ed.). *Rogers' Therapeutic Conditions: Evolution, Theory and Practice: Vol. 1. Congruence.* Ross-on-Wye, UK: PCCS Books.

Greenson, R. (1950). The mother-tongue of the mother. *The International Journal of Psychoanalysis,* 31: 18–23.

Griner, D., & Smith, T.B. (2006). Culturally adapted mental health interventions: A meta-analytic review. *Psychotherapy: Theory, research, practice, training,* 43(4): 531–548.

Guggenbuhl-Craig, A. (1979). *Power in the Helping Professions.* Irving, TX: Spring Publications.

Guttfreund, D.G. (1990). Effects of language usage on the emotional experience of Spanish-English and English-Spanish bilinguals. *Journal of Counselling and Clinical Psychology,* 58(5): 604–607.

Guy, J.D. (1987). *The Private Life of the Psychotherapist.* New York, NY: John Wiley & Sons.

Guy, J.D., & Liaboe, G. (1986). The impact of conducting psychotherapy upon interpersonal relationships of the psychotherapist. *Professional Psychology: Research and practice,* 17(2): 111–114.

Guy, J.D., Stark, M., & Polestra, P.L. (1987). National survey of psychotherapists' attitudes and beliefs. In J.D. Guy (Ed.). *The Private Life of the Psychotherapist.* New York, NY: John Wiley & Sons.

Hall, E., Hall, C., Harris, B., Hay, D., Biddulph, M., & Duffy, T. (1999). An evaluation of the long-term outcomes of small-group work for counsellor development. *British Journal of Guidance and Counselling*, 27(1): 99–112.

Harding-Davies, V., Alred, G., Hunt, K., & Davies, G. (2004). *Experiences of Counsellor Training: Challenge, surprise and change.* Basingstoke, UK: Palgrave MacMillan.

Harraway, D. (2003). *The Companion Species Manifesto: Dogs, people, and significant otherness.* Chicago, IL: Prickly Paradigm Press.

Harris, C.L., Gleason, J.B., & Avcucegi, A. (2006). When is a first language more emotional? Psychophysiological evidence from bilingual speakers. In A. Pavlenko (Ed.). *Bilingual Minds: Emotional experience, expression, and representation.* Clevedon, UK: Multilingual Matters.

Harvard Medical School (2006). Complicated grief; Looking for help when mourning persists and intensifies. *Harvard Mental Health Letter*, 23(4): 1–3.

Haugen, W.I. (1956). *Bilingualism in the Americas: A bibliography and research guide.* Tuscaloosa, AL: University of Alabama Press.

Haugh, S. (2012). A Person-Centred Approach to loss and bereavement. In J. Tolan, & P. Wilkins (Eds.). *Client Issues in Counselling and Psychotherapy.* London, UK: Sage Publications.

Hays, R.B. (1989). The day to day functioning of close versus casual friendships. *Journal of Social and Personal Relationships* 6: 21–37.

Helm, B.W. (2010). *Love, Friendship and the Self: Intimate identification and the sociality of persons.* Oxford, UK: Oxford University Press.

Henry, W.E., Sims, J.H., & Spray, S.L. (1973). *Public and Private Lives of Psychotherapists.* San Francisco, CA: Jossey-Bass.

Heredia, R.R., & Altarriba, J. (2001). Bilingual language mixing: Why do bilinguals code-switch? *Current Directions in Psychological Science*, 10(5): 164–168.

Hines, L.M. (2003). Historical perspectives on the human–animal bond. *The American Behavioral Scientist.* 47(1): 7–15.

Hirigoyen, M.-F. (1998). *Stalking the Soul: Emotional abuse and the erosion of identity.* Paris, France: La Decouverte and Syros.

Hochschild, A.R. (1983). *The Managed Heart: Commercialization of human feeling.* Berkeley, CA: University of California.

References

Hofberg, K., & Brockington, I. (2000). Tokophobia: An unreasoning dread of childbirth. *British Journal of Psychiatry,* 176: 83–85.

Hoffman, C. (1991). *An Introduction to Bilingualism,* London, UK: Longman.

Horley, S. (1991). *The Charm Syndrome: Why charming men can make dangerous lovers.* London, UK: Macmillan Publishers.

Horrocks, C., & Jevtic, Z. (1997). *Introducing Foucault.* New York, NY: Totem Books.

Howarth, R.A. (2011). Concepts and controversies in grief and loss. *Journal of Mental Health Counselling,* 33(1): 4–10.

Hoyle, A. (2013). *You're a Thick, Lazy, Useless Bitch. Nobody else would ever want you.* London, UK: IPC Media.

Humphrey, K.M. (2009). *Counseling Strategies for Loss and Grief.* Alexandria, VA: American Counseling Association.

Husserl, E. (1927). Phenomenology. *Encyclopaedia Britannica* (14th Edition). 17:699–702.

Iannaco, G. (2009). Wor(l)ds in translation: Mother-tongue and foreign language in psychodynamic practice. *Psychodynamic Practice,* 15(3): 261–274.

Imberti, P. (2007). Who resides behind the words? Exploring and understanding the language experience of the non-English-speaking immigrant. *Families in Society,* 88(1): 67–74.

Irvine, L. (2013). Animals as lifechangers and lifesavers: Pets in the redemption narratives of homeless people. *Journal of Contemporary Ethnography,* 42(3): 4–30.

Jacobs, S., & Prigerson, H. (2000). Psychotherapy of traumatic grief; A review of evidence for psychotherapeutic treatments. *Death Studies,* 24(6): 479–495.

James, K., & MacKinnon, L. (2010). The tip of the iceberg: A framework for identifying Non-Physical Abuse in couple and family relationships. *Journal of Feminist Family Therapy,* 22: 112–129.

Janoff-Bulman, R. (2004). Post-traumatic growth: Three explanatory models. *The Psychological Inquiry,* 15(1): 30–34.

Javier, R. (1989). Linguistic considerations in the treatment of bilinguals. *Psychoanalytic Psychology,* 6(1): 87–96.

Javier, R. (2007). *The Bilingual Mind*. New York, NY: Springer.

Javier, R.A. (1995). Vicissitudes of autobiographical memories in bilingual analysis. *Psychoanalytic Psychology,* 12(3): 429–438.

Jeffreys, J.S. (2005). *Helping Grieving People: When tears are not enough.* Abingdon, UK: Brunner-Routledge.

Johns, H. (1996). *Personal Development in Counsellor Training.* London, UK: Continuum.

Johnson, A.G. (2005). *The Gender Knot: Unravelling our patriarchal legacy.* Philadelphia, PA: Temple University Press.

Johnson, M. (2007). *The Meaning of the Body: Aesthetics of human understanding.* Chicago, IL: The University of Chicago.

Jones, G. (2007). Complimentary and psychological therapies in a rural hospital setting. *International Journal of Palliative Nursing,* 13(4): 184–189.

Jones, M. (1995). *Love After Death: Counselling in bereavement.* London, UK: Jessica Kingsley Publishers Ltd.

Joseph, S., & Butler, M. D. (2010). Positive changes following adversity. *PTSD Research Quarterly,* 21(3): 1–3.

Joseph, S., & Linley, P.A. (2005). Positive adjustment to threatening events: An organismic valuing theory of growth through adversity. *Review of General Psychology,* 9: 262–280.

Joseph, S., & Linley, P.A. (Ed.). (2008). *Trauma, Recovery and Growth.* Hoboken, NJ: John Wiley & Sons, Inc.

Jourard, S.M. (1971). *The Transparent Self.* New York, NY: Van Nostrand Reinhold.

Jung, C. (1951). The wounded healer. In D. Austin (Ed.). (2008). *The Theory and Practice of Vocal Psychotherapy: Songs of the self.* London, UK: Jessica Kingsley Publishers.

Karter, J. (2002). *On Training to be a Therapist: The long and winding road to qualification.* Milton Keynes, UK: Open University Press.

Katcher, A.H., & Beck, A. (Eds.). (1983). *New Perspectives on our Lives with Companion Animals.* Philadelphia, PA: University of Pennsylvania Press.

Kelly, G.A. (1955). *The Psychology of Personal Constructs. Volume one: A theory of personality.* New York, NY: Norton.

References

Kennedy, B.S.A. & Black, T.G. (2010). Life outside the fifty minute hour: The personal life of counsellors. *Canadian Journal of Counselling and Psychotherapy,* 44(4): 421–437.

King, G. (2008). Using counsellor supervision. In W. Dryden (Ed.). *Key Issues for Counselling in Action* (2nd Edition). London, UK: Sage Publications.

Kirchberg, T.M., Neimeyer, R.A., & James, R.K. (1998). Beginning counselors' death concerns and empathic responses to client situations involving death and grief. *Death Studies,* 22(2): 99–120.

Kirkwood, C. (1993). *Leaving Abusive Partners.* London, UK: Sage Publications.

Klesse, C. (2000). 'Modern Primitivism': Non-mainstream body modification and racialized representation. In M. Featherstone, *Body Modification.* London, UK: Sage Publications.

Klineberg, O. (1980). Historical perspectives: Cross-cultural psychology before 1960. In H.C. Triandis & W.W. Lambert (Eds.). *Handbook of Cross-Cultural Psychology.* Boston, MA: Allyn and Bacon.

Knapp, C. (1998). *Pack of Two: The intricate bond between people and dogs.* New York, NY: Dell Publishing.

Knight, S., & Herzog, H. (2009). All creatures great and small: New perspectives on psychology and human–animal interactions. *Journal of Social Issues,* 65(3): 451–461.

Kobak, R. (2009). Defining and measuring of attachment bonds: Comment on Kurdek. *Journal of Family Psychology,* 23(4): 447–449.

Kokaliari, E., Catanzarite, G., & Berzoff, J. (2013). It is called a mother-tongue for a reason: A qualitative study of therapists' perspectives on bilingual psychotherapy-treatment implications. *Smith College Studies in Social Work,* 83(1), 97–118.

Kosslyn, S.M., Alpert, N.M., Thompson, W.L., Maljkovic, V., Weise, S.B., Chabris, C.F., Hamilton, S.E., Rauch, S.L., & Buonanno, F.S. (1993). Visual mental imagery activates topographically organised visual cortex: PET investigations. *Journal of Cognitive Neuroscience,* 5(3): 263–287.

Kosut, M. (2000). Tattoo narratives: The intersection of the body, self-identity and society, *Visual Sociology*, 15: 79–100.

Kottler, J.A. (2010). *On Being a Therapist* (4th Edition). San Francisco, CA: Jossey-Bass.

Kubler-Ross, E. (1969). *On Death and Dying*. New York, NY: Scribner.

Kurdek, L. (2009). Pet dogs as attachment figures for adult owners. *Journal of Family Psychology*, 23: 439–446.

Kyriakopoulos, A.T. (2008). Grief, salutogenesis, rituals and counselling: A multidimensional framework for working with the bereaved. *European Journal of Psychotherapy and Counselling*, 10(4): 341–353.

Lachkar, J. (2000). Emotional abuse of high-functioning professional women: A psychodynamic perspective. *Journal of Emotional Abuse*, 2(1): 73–91.

Lamb, D.H. (1988). Loss and grief: Psychotherapy strategies and interventions. *Psychotherapy*, 25(4): 561–569.

Lammers, M., Richie, J., & Robertson, N. (2005). Women's experience of emotional abuse in intimate relationships: A qualitative study. *Journal of Emotional Abuse*, 5(1): 29–64.

Larcombe, A. (2008). Self-care in counselling. In W. Dryden, & A. Reeves (Eds.). *Key Issues for Counselling in Action* (2nd Edition). London, UK: Sage Publications.

Latham, A.E., & Prigerson, H.G. (2004). Suicidality and bereavement: Complicated grief as psychiatric disorder presenting greatest risk for suicidality. *Suicide and Life-Threatening Behavior*, 34(3): 350–362.

LeDoux, J. (1998). *The Emotional Brain*. New York, NY: Simon and Schuster.

Lemma, A. (2010). *Under the Skin: A psychoanalytic study of body modification*. London, UK: Routledge.

Lerner, H.G. (1989). *The Dance of Intimacy*. New York, NY: Harper and Row.

Levenson, B.M. (1969). *Pet Oriented Child Psychotherapy*. Springfield, IL: Charles C. Thomas.

References

Lewis, G. (2003). Addysg gynradd Gymraeg: Trochi a chyfoethogi disgyblion [Welsh primary education: Immersion and enrichment]. *The Welsh Journal of Education*, 12(2): 49–64.

Linley, P.A., & Joseph, S. (2004). Positive change following trauma and adversity: A review. *Journal of Traumatic Stress*, 17(1): 11–21.

Litsa. (2013, July 19). *Blog*. Retrieved August 30, 2013, from What's Your Grief?: http://whatsyourgrief.com/randos-six-r-processes-of-mourning/

Littell, A.E. (2003). The illustrated self: Construction of meaning through tattoo images and their narratives, *The Sciences and Engineering*, 64(1): 424.

Littlewood, J. (1992). *Aspects of Grief: Bereavement in adult life*. London, UK: Routledge.

Livingstone, A.G., Spears, R., Manstead, S.R., & Bruder, M. (2009). Illegitimacy and identity threat in (inter)action: Predicting intergroup orientations among minority group members. *British Journal of Social Psychology*, 48: 755–775.

Lorenz, K.Z. (2002). *Man Meets Dog*. London, UK: Routledge.

Loring, M.T. (1994). *Emotional Abuse: The trauma and treatment*. San Francisco, CA: Jossey-Bass Publishers.

Loring, M.T., & Powell, B. (1988). Gender, race, and DSM-111: A study of objectivity of psychiatric diagnostic behaviour. *Journal of Health and Social Behaviour*, 29: 1–22.

Love, A.W. (2007). Progress in understanding grief, complicated grief and caring for the bereaved. *Contemporary Nurse*, 27: 73–83.

Lupton, D. (1998). *The Emotional Self*. London, UK: Sage Publications.

Lynch, G. (2002). *Pastoral Care and Counselling*. London, UK: Sage Publications.

MacCallum, F., & Bryant, R.A. (2011). Imagining the future in complicated grief. *Depression and Anxiety*, 28: 658–665.

Machin, L. (2009). *Working with Loss & Grief*. London, UK: Sage Publications.

Maiello, S. (1997). Interplay: sound-aspects in mother-infant observation'. In S. Reid (Ed.). *Developments in Infant Observation: The Tavistock Model.* London, UK: Routledge.

Malcolm, J. (1980). *Psychoanalysis: The impossible profession.* New York, NY: Knopf.

Malim, T., Birch, A., & Wadeley, A. (1992). *Perspectives in Psychology.* Basingstoke, UK: Macmillan Press.

Mancini, A.J., Prati, G., & Bonanno, G.A. (2011). Do shattered world views lead to complicated grief? Prospective and longitudinal analyses. *Journal of Social and Clinical Psychology,* 30(2): 184–215.

Mander, G. (2004). The selection of candidates for training in psychotherapy and counselling. *Psychodynamic Practice,* 10(2): 161–172.

Marcos, L.R., (1976). Bilinguals in psychotherapy: Language as an emotional barrier. *American Journal of Psychotherapy,* 30: 552–559.

Marcos, L.R., & Alpert, M. (1976). Strategies and risks in psychotherapy with bilingual patients. *American Journal of Psychiatry,* 133: 1275–1278.

Marcos, L.R., & Urcuyo, L. (1979). Dynamic psychotherapy with the bilingual patient. *American Journal of Psychotherapy,* 33(3): 331–338.

Marian, V., & Neisser, U. (2000). Language dependent recall of autobiographical memories. *Journal of Experimental Psychology,* 129(3): 361–368.

Marshall, L.L. (1994). Physical and psychological abuse. In W.R. Cupach & B.H. Spitzberg (Eds.). *The Dark Side of Interpersonal Communication.* Hillsdale, NJ: Lawrence Erlbaum.

Marshall, L.L. (1996). Psychological abuse of women: Six distinct clusters. *Journal of Family Violence,* 11(4): 379–409.

Marwit, S.J. (1996). Reliability of diagnosing complicated grief: A preliminary investigation. *Journal of Consulting and Clinical Psychology,* 64(3): 563–568.

Maslow, A. (1943). A theory of human motivation. *Psychological Review,* 50(4): 370–396.

References

Maykut, P., & Morehouse, R. (1994). *Beginning Qualitative Research. A philosophical and practical guide.* London, UK: The Falmer Press.

McAucliffe, G.J. (2002). Student changes, programme influences and adult development in one programme of counsellor training: An exploratory inductive inquiry. *Journal of Adult Development,* 9(3): 205–216.

McDonald, M., & Wearing, S. (2013). A reconceptualisation of the self in humanistic psychology: Heidegger, Foucault and the sociocultural turn, *Journal of Phenomenological Psychology,* 44: 37–59.

McFarland, C., & Alvaro, C. (2000). The impact of motivation on temporal comparisons: Coping with traumatic events by perceiving personal growth. *Journal of Personality and Social Psychology,* 79: 327–343.

McGee, R., & Wolfe, D.A. (1991). Psychological maltreatment: Toward an operational definition. *Development and Psychopathology,* 3(1): 3–18.

McGrath, J., & Linley, A. (2006). Post-traumatic growth in acquired brain injury: A preliminary small-scale study. *Brain Injury,* 20: 767–773.

McLaren, J. (1998). A new understanding of grief: A counsellor's perspective. *Mortality,* 3(3): 275–290.

McLeod, J. (1993). *An Introduction to Counselling.* Milton Keynes, UK: Open University Press.

McLeod, J. (2009). *An Introduction to Counselling* (4th Edition). Maidenhead, UK: Open University Press.

McLeod, J. (2011). *Qualitative Research in Counselling and Psychotherapy* (2nd Edition). London, UK: Sage Publications.

McMillan, M. (2004). *The Person-Centred Approach to Theraputic Change.* London, UK: Sage Publications.

Mearns, D., (1997). *Person-Centred Counselling Training.* London, UK: Sage Publications.

Mearns, D. (2003). *Developing Person-Centred Counselling.* London, UK: Sage Publications.

Mearns, D., & Cooper, M. (2005). *Working at Relational Depth in Counselling and Psychotherapy*. London, UK: Sage Publications.

Mearns, D., & Thorne, B. (2000). *Person-Centred Therapy Today: New frontiers in theory and practice*. London, UK: Sage Publications.

Mearns, D., & Thorne, B. (2013). *Person-Centred Counselling in Action* (4th Edition). London, UK: Sage Publications.

Merry, T. (2002). *Learning and Being in Person-Centred Counselling* (2nd Edition). Ross-on-Wye, UK: PCCS Books.

Mezey, N.J., Post, L.A., & Maxwell, C.D., (2002). Redefining intimate partner violence: Women's experiences with physical violence and non-physical abuse by age. *International Journal of Sociology and Social Policy*, 22(7): 122–154.

Mezirow, J. (2000). *Learning as Transformation: Critical perspectives on a theory in progress*. San Francisco, CA: Jossey Bass.

Miliora, M.T. (1998). Trauma, dissociation, and somatization: A self-psychology perspective, *Journal of the American Academy of Psychoanalysis,* 26(2): 273–293.

Miller, G.D., & Baldwin Jr, D.C. (2013). The implications of the wounded-healer archetype of the use of self in psychotherapy. In M. Baldwin (Ed.). *The Use of Self in Therapy* (3rd Edition). Hove, UK: Routledge.

Miller, J. (2006). A specification of the types of intimate partner violence experienced by women in the general population. *Violence against Women*, 12(12): 1105–1131.

Miller, J.B. (1976/1986). *Towards a New Psychology of Women*. Boston, MA: Beacon Press.

Miller, J.B., & Stiver, I.P. (1997). *The Healing Connection: How women form relationships in Therapy and in Life*. Boston, MA: Beacon Press.

Miller, M.S. (1995). *No Visible Wounds: Identifying non-physical abuse of women by their men*. New York, NY: Random House.

Mohr, C.M., & Barner, J.R. (2012). Prevalence of partner abuse: Rates of emotional abuse and control. *Partner Abuse*, 3(3): 286–335.

Moerier, D., Bryan, A.E.B., & Kasdin, L. (2011). The effects of group identity, group choice, and strength of group identification on intergroup sensitivity, *Group Dynamics: Theory, research, and practice,* 17(1): 14–29.

Muggleton, D. (1995). From 'Subculture' to 'Neo-Tribe': Identity, paradox and postmodernism' in 'Alternative Style'. Unpublished paper presented at 'Shouts from the Street: Culture, Creativity and Change', MIPC Conference on Popular Culture, Manchester Metropolitan University, September.

Muldoon, M.S. (2006). *Tricks of Time: Bergson, Merleau-Ponty and Ricoeur in search of time, self and meaning.* Pittsburgh, PA: Duquesne University Press.

Mullally, S.M. (2000). Shame and trauma correlates of emotional abuse among women in partnered relationships. *Dissertation Abstracts International,* 61(1–B): 542.

Muller, E.D., & Thompson, C.L. (2003). The experience of grief after bereavement: A phenomenological study with implications for mental health counseling. *Journal of Mental Health Counseling,* 25(3): 183–203.

Murray, L., Fiori-Cowley, A., & Hooper, R. (1996). The impact of postnatal depression and associated adversity on early mother-infant interactions and later infant outcome. *Child Development,* 67: 2512–2526.

Nangle, D.W., Erdley, C.A., Newman, J.E., Mason, C.A. & Carpenter, E.M. (2003). Popularity, friendship quantity and friendship quality: Interactive influences on children's loneliness and depression. *Journal of Clinical Child and Adolescent Psychology,* 32: 546–555.

Natiello, P. (2001). *The Person-Centred Approach: A passionate presence.* Ross-on-Wye, UK: PCCS Books.

National Assembly for Wales (2003). *Iaith Pawb: A national action plan for a bilingual Wales.* National Assembly for Wales, Cardiff, UK: 47.

Neimeyer, R.A. (2001). *Meaning Reconstruction and the Experience of Loss.* Washington, DC: American Psychological Association.

Neimeyer, R.A., Prigerson, H.G., & Davies, B. (2002). Mourning and meaning. *The American Behavioural Scientist,* 46(2): 235–251.

Newson, R.S., Boelan, P.A., Hek, K., Hofman, A., & Tiemeir, H. (2011). The prevalence and characteristics of complicated grief in older adults. *Journal of Affective Disorders*, 132: 231–238.

Nichols, K., & Ayers, S. (2007). Childbirth-related post-traumatic stress disorder in couples: A qualitative study. *British Journal of Health Psychology*, 12: 491–509.

Nijenhuis, E., Van Engen, A., Kusters, I., & Van der Hart, O. (2001). Peritraumatic somatoform and psychological dissociation in relation to recall of childhood sexual abuse. *Journal of Trauma and Dissociation*, 2(3): 49–68.

Noonan, E. (2008). People and pets. *Psychodynamic Practice*, 4(14): 395–407.

Ober, A.M., Granello, D.H., & Wheaton, J.E. (2012). Grief counseling: An investigation of counselors' training, experience, and competencies. *Journal of Counseling and Development*, 90: 150–159.

Odendaal, J. (2002). *Pets and Our Mental Health: The why, the what, and the how.* New York, NY: Vantage Press.

O'Driscoll, M. (1994). Midwives, childbirth and sexuality. *British Journal of Midwifery*, 2: 39–41.

O'Hagan, K.P. (1995). Emotional and psychological abuse: Problems of definition. *Child Abuse and Neglect*, 19(4): 449–461.

O'Hagan, K.P. (2006). *Identifying Emotional and Psychological Abuse. A guide for childcare professionals.* Maidenhead, UK: Open University Press.

Olde E., Van der Hart, O., Kleber, R., & Van Son, M. (2006). Posttraumatic stress following childbirth: A review. *Clinical Psychology Review*, 26: 1–16.

Omylinska-Thurston, J., & James, P.E. (2011). The therapist's use of self: A closer look at the processes within congruence. *Counselling Psychology Review*, 26(3): 20–33.

Orlinsky, D.E. (2012). The psychotherapeutic relationship, personal life and modern culture. *Tidsskrift for Norsk Psykologforening.* 49(5): 442–449.

References

Outlaw, M. (2009). No one type of intimate partner abuse: Exploring physical and non-physical abuse among intimate partners. *Journal of Family Violence*, 24: 263–272.

Owen, I. (1993). On the private life of the psychotherapist and the psychology of caring. *Counselling and Psychology Quarterly*, 6(3): 251–264.

Owen, J. (2008). A blue tit got me thinking … Reflections on the therapeutic aspects of human–animal relationships. *Counselling Psychological Review*, 23(2): 47–52.

Paradis, M. (2008). Bilingualism and neuropsychiatric disorders. *Journal of Neurolinguistics*, 21(3): 199–230.

Parahoo, K. (1997). *Nursing Research. Principles, Process and Issues*. Basingstoke, UK: Palgrave Macmillan.

Parfitt, Y.M., & Ayers, S. (2009). The effect of post-natal symptoms of post-traumatic stress and depression on the couple's relationship and parent–baby bond. *Journal of Reproductive and Infant Psychology*, 27(2): 127–142.

Park, C., (2010). Making sense of the meaning literature: An integrative review of meaning making and its effects on adjustment to stressful life events. *Psychological Bulletin, American Psychological Association,* 136(2): 257–301.

Park, C.L., & Helgeson, V.S. (2006). Growth following highly stressful life events: Current status and future directions. *Journal of Consulting and Clinical Psychology*, 74: 791–796.

Parkes, C.M., & Prigerson, H.G. (2010). *Bereavement: Studies in adult life*. London, UK: Penguin.

Patton, W., & Mannison, M. (1995). Sexual coercion in high school dating. *Sex Roles*, 33: 447–457.

Patterson, M., & Schroeder, D. (2010). Borderlines: Skin, tattoos and consumer culture theory. *UK Marketing Theory*, 10(3): 253–267.

Pattison, S., Rowland, N., Richards, K., Cromarty, K., Jenkins, P., & Polat, F. (2009). School counselling in Wales: Recommendations for good practice. *Counselling and Psychotherapy Research*, 9(3): 169–173.

Pavlenko, A. (2008). Emotion and emotion-laden words in the bilingual lexicon. *Bilingualism: Language and cognition*, 11(2): 146–164.

Payne, S., Jarrett, N., Wiles, R., & Field, D. (2002). Counselling strategies for bereaved people offered in primary care. *Counselling Psychology Quarterly*, 15(2): 161–177.

Peacock, J., Chur-Hansen, A., & Winefield, H. (2012). Mental health implications of human attachment to companion animals. *Journal of Clinical Psychology*, 68(3): 292–303.

Peeler, S., Stedmon, J., & Skirton, H. (2013). A review assessing the current treatment strategies for postnatal psychological morbidity with a focus on post-traumatic stress disorder. *Midwifery*, 29: 377–388.

Perez-Foster, R. (1996). The bilingual self: Duet in two voices. *Psychoanalytic Dialogues*, 6(1): 99–121.

Perez-Foster, R. (1998). *The Power of Language in the Clinical Process: Assessing and treating the bilingual person*. North Bergen, NJ: Jason Aronson.

Phelps, K.A., Miltenberger, R.G., Jens. T., & Wadeson, H. (2008). An investigation of the effects of dog visits on depression, mood, and social interaction in elderly individuals living in a nursing home. *Behavioral Interventions*, 23(3): 181–200.

Philippe, F.L., Koestner, R., Lecours, S., Beaulieu-Pelletier, G., & Bois, K. (2011). The role of autobiographical memory networks in the experience of negative emotions: How our remembered past elicits our current feelings. *Emotion*, 11(6): 1279–1290.

Pitts, V. (2003). *In the Flesh: The cultural politics of body modification*. New York, NY: Palgrave MacMillan.

Podberscek, A., Paul, E., & Serpell, J. (Eds.). (2000). *Companion Animals and Us*. Cambridge, UK: Cambridge University Press.

Polkinghorne, D. (2001). The self and humanistic psychology. In K.J. Schneider, J.F.T. Bugental, & J.F. Pierson (Eds.). *The Handbook of Humanistic Psychology: Leading edges in theory, research and practice*. Thousand Oaks, CA: Sage Publications.

Power, C. (2004). Romantic love and domestic violence. *Australian Nursing Journal*, 11(8): 36.

References

Prigerson, H. (2004). Complicated grief: When the path of adjustment leads to a dead-end. *Bereavement Care,* 23(3): 38–40.

Prigerson, H.G., Bierhals, A.J., Kasl, S.V., Reynolds III, C.F., Shear, M.K., Newsom, J.T., & Jacobs, S. (1996). Complicated grief as a disorder distinct from bereavement-related depression and anxiety: A replication study. *The American Journal of Psychiatry,* 53(11): 1484–1486.

Prigerson, H.G., & Maciejewski, P.K. (2006). A call for empirical testing and evaluation of criteria for complicated grief proposed for DSM-V. *Omega,* 52(1): 9–19.

Proctor, G. (2002). *The Dynamics of Power in Counselling and Psychotherapy: Ethics, politics and practice.* Ross-on-Wye, UK: PCCS Books.

Puterbaugh, D.T. (2008). Spiritual evolution of bereavement counselors: An exploratory qualitative study. *Counseling and Values,* 52: 198–210.

Ramos-Sanchez, L. (2007). Language switching and Mexican Americans' emotional expression. *Journal of Multicultural Counselling and Development,* 35: 154–167.

Ramos-Sanchez, L. (2009). Counselor bilingual ability, counselor ethnicity, acculturation, and Mexican Americans' perceived counselor credibility. *Journal of Counseling and Development,* 87: 311–318.

Rando, T.A. (2013). On achieving clarity regarding complicated grief: Lessons from clinical practice. In M. Strobe, H. Schut, & J. van den Bout (Eds.). *Complicated Grief: Scientific foundations for healthcare professionals.* Hove, UK: Routledge.

Rando, T.A., Doka, K.J., Fleming, S., Franco, M.H., Lobb, E.A., Murray Parkes, C., & Steele, R. (2012). A call to the field: Complicated grief in the DSM-5. *Omega,* 65(4): 251–255.

Reed, G.L., & Enright, R.D. (2006). The effects of forgiveness therapy on depression, anxiety and posttraumatic stress for women after spousal emotional abuse. *Journal of Consulting and Clinical Psychology,* 74(5): 920–929.

Reid, M. (2011). The impact of traumatic delivery on the mother-infant relationship. *Infant Observation,* 14(2): 117–128.

Rennie, D.L. (1998). *Person-Centred Counselling: An experiential approach.* London, UK: Sage Publications.

Reynolds, J.L. (1997). Post-traumatic stress disorder after childbirth: The phenomenon of traumatic birth. *Canadian Medical Association Journal,* 156(6): 831–835.

Riessman, C.K. (2000). *Analysis of Personal Narratives.* Boston, MA: Boston University Press.

Rippere, V. & Williams, R. (1985). *Wounded Healers: Mental health workers' experiences of depression.* New York, NY: Wiley.

Ro, E., & Lawrence, E. (2007). Comparing three measures of psychological aggression: Psychometric properties and differentiation from negative communication. *Journal of Family Violence,* 22: 575–586.

Robinson, I. (1995). *The Waltham Book of Human–animal Interaction.* Oxford, UK: Pergamon.

Rogers, C. (1957). The necessary and sufficient conditions of therapeutic personality change, *Journal of Consulting Psychology,* 21(2): 95–103.

Rogers, C. (1961). *On Becoming a Person: A therapist's view of Psychotherapy.* London, UK: Constable.

Rogers, C.R. (1951). *Client-Centred Therapy: Its current practice, implications and theory.* Boston, MA: Houghton Mifflin Company.

Rogers, C.R. (1979). *Foundations.* Retrieved August 30, 2013, from Elements UK: http://www.elementsuk.com/libraryofarticles/foundations.pdf

Rogers, C.R. (1980). *A Way of Being.* New York, NY: Houghton Mifflin Company.

Ronnestad, M.H., & Skovholt, T.M. (2003). The journey of the counsellor and therapist: Research findings and perspectives on professional development. *Journal of Career Development,* 30(1): 5–44.

Rose, C. (2012). Self awareness in psychotherapy and counselling. In C. Rose (Ed.). *Self Awareness and Personal Development Resources for Psychotherapists and Counsellors.* Basingstoke, UK: Palgrave Macmillan.

References

Rose, C., & Worsley, R. (2012). Thinking about the Self. In C. Rose (Ed.). *Self Awareness and Personal Development: Resources for psychotherapists and counsellors.* Basingstoke, UK: Palgrave Macmillan.

Rosenblatt, P.C. (2013). The concept of complicated grief: Lesson from other cultures. In M. Stroebe, H. Schut, & J. van den Bout (Eds.). *Complicated Grief: Scientific foundations for healthcare professionals.* Hove, UK: Routledge.

Rowan, A.N. (Ed.). (1988). *Animals and People Sharing the World.* Hanover, NH: University Press of New England.

Rozensky, R.H., & Gomez, M.Y. (1983). Language switching in psychotherapy with bilinguals: Two problems, two models, and case examples. *Psychotherapy: Therapy, Research and Practice*, 20: 152–160.

Rubin, S.S., Malkinson, R., & Witztum, E. (2012). *Working with the Bereaved: Multiple lenses on loss and mourning.* New York, NY: Routledge.

Russell, J., & Dexter, G. (2008). *Blank Mind and Sticky Moments in Counselling: Practical strategies and provocative themes.* London, UK: Sage Publications.

Ryding, E.L., Wijma, K., & Wijma, B. (1998). Experiences of emergency caesarean section: A phenomenological study of 53 women. *Birth*, 25: 246–251.

Sable, P. (2013). The pet connection: An attachment perspective. *Clinical Social Work Journal,* 41: 93–99.

Sackett, L.A., & Saunders, D.G. (1999). The impact of different forms of psychological abuse on battered women. *Violence and Victims*, 14: 105–117.

Samuel, S.A. (2011). An examination of the psychological role of tattoos in mourning. *Dissertations Abstracts International: Section B: The Sciences and Engineering,* 72(1–B): 553.

Sanders, C., & Vail, D. (2008). *Customising the Body: The art and culture of tattooing.* Philadelphia, PA: Temple University Press.

Sanders, P., & Wilkins, P. (2010). *First Steps in Practitioner Research.* Ross-on-Wye, UK: PCCS Books Ltd.

Santiago-Rivera, A.L. (1995). Developing a culturally sensitive treatment modality for bilingual Spanish-speaking clients: Incorporating language and culture in counselling. *Journal of Counseling and Development*, 74: 12–17.

Santiago-Rivera, A.L., & Altarriba, J. (2002). The role of language in therapy with the Spanish-English bilingual client. *Professional Psychology: Research and practice*, 33(1): 30–38.

Santiago-Rivera, A.L., Altarriba, J., Poll, N., Gonzalez-Miller, N., & Cragun, C. (2009). Therapists' views on working with bilingual Spanish-English speaking clients: A qualitative investigation. *Professional Psychology: Research and practice*, 40(5): 436–443.

Satir, V. (2013). The therapist story. In M. Baldwin (Ed.). *The Use of Self in Therapy* (3rd Edition). Hove, UK: Routledge.

Sawyer, A., & Ayers, S. (2009). Post-traumatic growth in women after childbirth, *Psychology and Health,* 24(4): 457–471.

Sawyer, A., Ayers, S., Young, D., Bradley, R., & Smith, H. (2012). Posttraumatic growth after childbirth: A prospective study. *Psychology and Health,* 27(3): 362–377.

Sarnecki, J.H. (2001). Trauma and tattoo. *Anthropology of Consciousness,* 12(2): 35–42.

Schwab, J.R., & Frances, L. (2013). Religious meaning making: Positioning identities through stories, *Psychology of Religion and Spirituality,* 5(3): 219–226.

Seashore, C. (1995). In grave danger of growing. *Social Change,* 5(4): 1–4.

Seff, L.R., Beaulaurier, R.L., & Newman, F.L. (2008). Nonphysical abuse: Findings in domestic violence against older women study. *Journal of Emotional Abuse,* 8(3): 355–374.

Segalowitz, N., (1976). Communicative incompetence and the non-fluent bilingual. *Canadian Journal of Behavioural Sciences,* 8: 122–125.

Segrott, J. (2001). Language, geography and identity: The case of the Welsh in London. *Social and Cultural Geography,* 2(3): 281–296.

Serpell, J. (1995). *The Domestic Dog: Its evolution, behaviour and interactions with people.* Cambridge, UK: Cambridge University Press.

References

Serpell, J. (1998). *In the Company of Animals*. Cambridge, UK: Cambridge University Press.

Serpell, J.A. (2002). Anthropomorphism and anthropomorphic selection—beyond the 'cute response'. *Society and Animals*, 10(4): 437–454.

Servaty-Seib, H.L. (2004). Connections between counseling theories and current theories of grief and mourning. *Journal of Mental Health Counseling*, 26(2): 125–145.

Shanahan, D. (2008). A new view of language, emotion, and the brain. *Integrated Psychology and Behaviour*, 42: 6–19.

Shear, K.M. (2012). Grief and mourning gone awry: Pathway and course of complicated grief, *Dialogues in Clinical Neuroscience*, 14(2): 119–128.

Shear, K.M., & Mulhare, E. (2008). Complicated grief. *Psychiatric Annals*, 38: 662–670.

Shear, K.M., Simon, N., Wall, M., Zisook, S., Neimeyer, R., & Duan, N. (2001). Complicated grief and bereavement issues for DSM-5. *Depression and Anxiety*, 28(2): 103–117.

Sheldrake, R. (2000). *Dogs That Know When Their Owners Are Coming Home*. London, UK: Arrow Books.

Shilling, C. (1993). *The Body and Social Theory*, London, UK: Sage Publications.

Shmotkin, D., & Eyal, N. (2003). Psychological time in later life: Implications for counseling. *Journal of Counseling and Development*, 81: 259–276.

Siegel, J.M. (1990). Stressful life events and use of physician services among the elderly: Moderating role of pet ownership. *Journal of Personality and Social Psychology*, 58(6): 1081–1086.

Siegel, J.M. (1993). Companion animals: In sickness and in health. *Journal of Social Issues*, 49(1): 157–167.

Silverman, D. (2010). *Qualitative Research* (3rd Edition). London, UK: Sage Publications.

Silverman, P.R., & Klass, D. (1996). Introduction: What's the problem? In D. Klass, P.R. Silverman, & S.L. Nickman (Eds.). *Continuing Bonds: New understandings of grief*. Philadelphia, PA: Taylor & Francis.

Simon, N.M. (2012). Is complicated grief a post-loss stress disorder? *Depression and Anxiety*, 29: 541–544.

Sims, C.-D.L. (2008). Invisible wounds, invisible abuse: The exclusion of emotional abuse in newspaper articles. *Journal of Emotional Abuse*, 8(4): 375–402.

Skovholt, T.M., & Ronnestad, M.H. (1992). *The Evolving Professional Self: Stages and themes in professional counsellor development*. New York, NY: John Wiley & Sons.

Smith, J., & Osborn, M. (1998). The personal experience of chronic benign lower back pain: An interpretative phenomenological analysis. *British Journal of Health Psychology*, 3: 65–83.

Smith, J.A., Flowers, P., & Larkin, M. (2009). *Interpretative Phenomenological Analysis: Theory, method and research*. London, UK: Sage Publications.

Society for Companion Animal Studies (2013a). *Terminology*. Retrieved from http://www.scas.org.uk/1849/terminology.html

Society for Companion Animal Studies (2013b). *Benefits of the Bond*. Retrieved from http://www.scas.org.uk/1851/benefits-of-the-bond.html

Soet, J.E., Brack, G.A., & Dilorio, C. (2003). Prevalence and predictors of women's experience of psychological trauma during childbirth. *Birth*, 30: 36–46.

Sorsoli, L. (2004). Hurt feeling: Emotional abuse and the failure of empathy. *Journal of Emotional Abuse*, 4(1): 110–128.

Souza, P., Cecatti, J.G., Parpinelli, M., Krupa, F., & Osis, M. (2009). An emerging 'maternal near-miss syndrome': Narratives of women who almost died during pregnancy and childbirth. *Birth*, 36(2): 149–158.

Speigel, P.B. (1990). Confidentiality endangered under some circumstances without special management, *Psychotherapy*, 27: 636–643.

Spinelli, E. (2005). *The Interpreted World: An introduction to phenomenological psychology*. London, UK: Sage Publications.

References

Sprang, G., & McNeil, J. (1995). *The Many Faces of Bereavement: The nature and treatment of natural, traumatic and stigmatized grief.* New York, NY: Brunner/Mazel, Inc.

Sprowls, C. (2002). Bilingual therapists' perspectives of their language related self-experience during therapy. *Dissertation Abstracts International,* 63(04) 2076B. UMI No. 3052139.

Staats, S., Sears, K., & Pierfelice, L. (2006). Teachers' pets and why have them: An investigation of the human animal bond. *Journal of Applied Social Psychology,* 36(8): 1881–1891.

Stark. E. (2007). *Coercive Control: How men entrap women in personal life.* New York, NY: Oxford University Press.

Stern, D. (1998). *The Interpersonal World of the Infant,* London, UK: Karnac.

Stevens, R. (1996). *Understanding the Self.* London, UK: Sage Publications.

Stewart, C.S., Thrush, J.C., & Paulus, G. (1989). Disenfranchised bereavement and loss of a companion animal: Implications for caring communities. In K. J. Doka (Ed.). *Disenfranchised Grief.* Lexington, KY: Lexington Books.

Strang, P. (2000). Qualitative research methods in palliative medicine and palliative oncology. *Acta Oncologica,* 39(8): 911–917.

Stroebe, M., & Schut, H. (1999). The dual process model of coping with bereavement: Rationale and description. *Death Studies,* 23(3): 197–224.

Sussman, M.B. (1992). *A Curious Calling.* Northvale, NJ: Jason Aronson.

Sutton, T.M., Altarriba, J., Gianico, J.L., & Basnight-Brown, D.M. (2007). The automatic access of emotion: Emotional Stroop effects in Spanish-English bilingual speakers. *Cognition and Emotion,* 21(5): 1077–1090.

Tamura, L.J., Guy, J.D., Brady, J.L., & Grace, C. (1996). Maintaining confidentiality, avoiding burnout and psychotherapists' needs for inclusion: A national survey. *Psychotherapy in Private Practice,* 13(2): 1–17.

313

Taylor, S.E., Kemeny, M.E., Reed, G.F., Bower, J.E., & Gruenewald, T.L. (2000). Psychological resources, positive illusions, and health. *American Psychologist*, 55: 99–109.

Tedeschi, R.G., Park, C.L., & Calhoun L.G. (1998). Posttraumatic growth; conceptual issues. In R.G. Tedeschi, C.L. Park, & L.G. Calhoun (Eds.). *Posttraumatic Growth: Positive changes in the aftermath of crisis*. Mahwah, NJ: Lawrence Erlbaum Associates, Publishers.

Tedeschi, R.G., Park, C.L., & Calhoun, L.G. (2004). Posttraumatic growth: Conceptual foundations and empirical evidence. *Psychology Inquiry*, 15: 1–18.

Tehrani, N., & Vaughan, S. (2009). Lost in translation: Using bilingual differences to increase emotional mastery following bullying. *Counselling and Psychotherapy Research*, 9(1): 11–17.

Tennen, H., & Affleck, G. (2002). Benefit-finding and benefit reminding. In C.R. Snyder & S.J. Lopez (Eds.). *Handbook of Positive Psychology*. Oxford, UK: Oxford University Press.

Terkel, S. (1972). *Working: People talk about what they do all day and how they feel about what they do*. New York, NY: The New Press.

Terr, L.C. (1991). Childhood traumas: An outline and overview. *American Journal of Psychiatry*, 148(1): 10–19.

Therriault, A., & Gazzola, N. (2008). Feelings of incompetence in therapy: Causes, consequences and coping strategy. In W. Dryden (Ed.). (2nd Edition). *Key Issues for Counselling in Action*. London, UK: Sage Publications.

Thompson, A., & Day, G. (1999). Situating Welshness: 'Local' experience and national identity. In R. Fevre & A. Thompson (Eds.). *National Identity and Social Theory: Perspectives from Wales*. Cardiff, UK: University of Wales Press.

Thomson, G., & Downe, S. (2008). Widening the trauma discourse: The link between childbirth and experiences of abuse. *Journal of Psychosomatic Obstetrics and Gynaecology*, 29(4): 268–273.

Thomson, G., & Downe, S. (2010). Changing the future to change the past: Women's experiences of a positive birth following a traumatic birth experience. *Journal of Reproductive and Infant Psychology*, 28(1): 102–112.

314

References

Thorenson, R.W., Miller, M., & Krauskopf, C.J. (1989). The distressed psychologist: Prevalence and treatment considerations, *Professional Psychology: Research and Practice,* 20: 153–158.

Tjaden, P., & Thoennes, N. (2000). *Extent, Nature, and Consequences of Intimate Partner Violence: Findings from the national violence against women survey.* Rockville, MD: National Institute of Justice.

Tolman, R.M. (1989). The development of a measure of psychological maltreatment of women by their male partners. *Violence and Victims,* 4(3): 159–177.

Truell, R. (2001). The stresses of learning counselling: Six recent graduates comment on their personal experience of learning counselling and what can be done to reduce associated harm. *Counselling Psychology Quarterly,* 24(2): 67–89.

Tummala-Narra, P. (2001). Asian trauma survivors: Immigration identity loss and recovery. *Journal of Psychoanalytic Studies,* 3(3): 243–258.

Turner, B.S. (2000). The possibility of primitiveness: Towards a sociology of body marks in cool societies. In M. Featherstone, (Ed.). *Body Modification.* London, UK: Sage Publications.

Verdinelli, S., & Biever, J.L. (2009). Spanish-English bilingual psychotherapists: Personal and professional language development and use. *Cultural Diversity and Ethnic Minority Psychology,* 15(3): 230–242.

Verdinelli, S., & Biever, J.L. (2013). Therapists' experiences of cross-ethnic therapy with Spanish-speaking Latina/o Clients. *Journal of Latina/o Psychology,* 1(4): 227–242.

Vining, J. (2003). The connection to other animals and caring for nature. *Human Ecology Review,* 10(2): 87–99.

Walsh, F. (2009a). Human–animal bonds I: The relational significance of companion animals. *Family Process,* 48(4): 462–480.

Walsh, F. (2009b). Human–animal bonds II: The role of pets in family systems and family therapy. *Family Process,* 48(4): 481–499.

Wells, D. (2011). The value of pets for human health. *The Psychologist,* 24(3): 172–176.

Welsh Assembly Government (2012a). Together for mental health: A strategy for mental health and wellbeing in Wales. (http://wales.gov.uk/docs/dhss/publications/121031tmhfin alen.pdf). Accessed January 9, 2013.

Welsh Assembly Government (2012b). More than Just Words: Strategic Framework for Welsh Language Services in Health, Social Services, and Social Care. The Welsh Government Consultation Document. (http://wales.gov.uk/docs/dhss/consultation/120208welshlangstrategicframeworken.pdf). Accessed January 9, 2013.

West, W. (2011). Using the tacit dimension in qualitative research in counselling psychology. *Counselling Psychology Review,* 26(4): 40–45.

Wheeler, S. (2002). Nature or nurture: Are therapists born or trained? *Psychodynamic Practice,* 8: 427–441.

Wheeler-Roy, S., & Amyot, B.A. (2004). *Grief Counseling Resource Guide; A field manual.* Retrieved July 13, 2013, from New York State Office of Mental Health: http://www.omh.ny.gov/omhweb/grief/Grief CounselingResourceGuide.pdf

White, M. (2007). *Maps of Narrative Practice.* London, UK: W.W. Norton and Company.

White, T., Matthey, S., Boyd, K., & Barnett, B. (2006). Postnatal depression and post-traumatic stress after childbirth: Prevalence, course and co-occurrence. *Journal of Reproductive and Infant Psychology,* 24(2): 107–120.

Whorf, B.L. (1950). An American-Indian model of the universe. *International Journal of American Linguistics,* 16: 67–72.

Wijma, K., Soderquist, J., & Wijma, B. (1997). Posttraumatic stress disorder after childbirth: A cross-sectional study. *Journal of Anxiety Disorders,* 11: 587–597.

Wilkins, P. (1999). The relationship in person-centred counselling. In C. Feltham, (Ed.). *Understanding the Counselling Relationship.* London, UK: Sage Publications.

References

Williams, D.I. & Irving, J.A. (1996). Personal Growth: Rogerian paradoxes. *British Journal of Guidance and Counselling*, 24(2): 165–172.

Willig, C. (2008). *Introducing Qualitative Research in Psychology* (3rd Edition). New York, NY: McGraw-Hill International.

Wittouck, C., Van Autreve, S., De Jaegere, E., Portzky, G., & van Heeringen, K. (2011). The prevention and treatment of complicated grief: A meta-analysis. *Clinical Psychology Review*, 31: 69–78.

Wood, L.J., Giles-Corti, B., Bulsara, M.K., & Borsch, D.A. (2007). More than a furry companion: The ripple effect of companion animals of neighbourhood interactions and sense of community. *Society and Animal*, 15(1): 43–56.

Woods, S. (1999). Normative beliefs regarding the maintenance of intimate relationships among abused and non-abused women. *Journal of Interpersonal Violence*, 14: 479–491.

Worden, J.W. (2010). *Grief Counselling and Grief Therapy* (4th Edition). Hove, UK: Routledge.

Wortman, C.B., & Cohen Silver, R. (1989). The myths of coping with loss. *Journal of Consulting and Clinical Psychology*, 57(3): 349–357.

Worsley, R. (2008). Lived experience. *Therapy Today*, 19(1): 14–17.

Wright, C. (2004). Counselling training and its effect on personal relationships and friendships – all change here? *Healthcare Counselling and Psychotherapy Journal*, 4(3): 41–43.

Wylie, L., Hollinsmartin, C.J., Marland, G., Martin, C.R., & Rankin, J. (2011). The enigma of post-natal depression: An update. *Journal of Psychiatric and Mental Health Nursing*, 18: 48–58.

Yariv, G. (1999). Eternity in an hour: Experiences of time related to psychotherapy sessions. *Journal of Analytical Psychology*, 44: 37–55.

Zimmer, C. (2011). *Science Ink: Tattoos of the science obsessed*. New York, NY: Sterling.

Zink, T., Regan, S., Jacobson, C.J., & Pabst, S. (2003). Cohort, period and aging effects: A qualitative study of older women's reasons for remaining in abusive relationships. *Violence Against Women*, 9: 1429–1441.